DATES IN
UROLOGY

DATES IN

UROLOGY

EDITED BY H.S.J. LEE

The Parthenon Publishing Group
International Publishers in Medicine, Science & Technology

NEW YORK   LONDON

Library of Congress Cataloging-in-Publication Data

Dates in urology / edited by H.S.J.Lee.
    p. cm. -- (Landmarks in medicine series, ISSN 1467-7253)
  ISBN 1-85070-496-1 (alk paper)
  1. Urology -- History. I. Lee, H. S. J. II. Series
  [DNLM: 1. Urology -- Chronology. WJ 11. 1 D232 1999]
  RG870.8. D38 1999
  616.6'009--dc21   99-055487

British Library Cataloguing in Publication Data

Dates in urology. - (Landmarks in medicine series)
    1. Urology - History - Chronology
    I. Lee, H. S. J
 616.6'009

  ISBN 1-85070-496-1

Published in the USA by
The Parthenon Publishing Group Inc.
One Blue Hill Plaza
PO Box 1564, Pearl River
New York 10965, USA

Published in the UK and Europe by
The Parthenon Publishing Group Limited
Casterton Hall, Carnforth
Lancs. LA6 2LA, UK

Printed and bound by Bookcraft (Bath) Ltd., Midsomer Norton, UK

Acknowledgment

The editor would like to acknowledge the National Library of Medicine, World Health Organization and the Nobel Foundation.

Introduction

Modern understanding of urology is based on the achievements and contributions of many doctors and scientists over many years. To appreciate the state-of-the-art as it exists today, it is helpful to know something of the background and history of the subject as it has developed over the last few centuries – and as the underlying scientific principles have become more fully understood and elucidated.

This volume records some of the key milestones in the development of modern urology that have taken place over the millennium. Of course, although some notable contributions were made in earlier centuries, it is really only in the later years of the present millennium that advances in knowledge and practice become numerous and significant. Naturally, too, these advances are closely related to progress in other fields of medicine – and this fact is also reflected in the pages of the book.

The milestones listed here are indeed important ones but are by no means comprehensive. Readers will all have their own individual views of additional important events that should be recorded, and I would certainly welcome their suggestions for the next edition.

It is hoped that the milestones described will provide an interesting reference and aide-memoire to all those with an interest in urology who would like to know more about its background and development. At the start of the new millennium it seems appropriate to look back and chart the dramatic progress that has been made in the course of the preceding one.

c. 1500 BC   The Ebers Papyrus was written. A systematic classification of remedies and medicines used in ancient Egypt. It records the use of 'bread in a rotten condition' to treat bladder diseases.

460 BC   HIPPOCRATES born.
He recognized the dangers of bladder stones and initiated the analysis of urine by inspection and tasting.

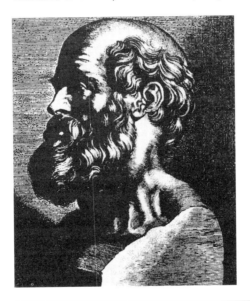

Hippocrates
(460–377)

372 BC   THEOPHRASTUS born.
A Greek physician and philosopher who wrote several treatises including *Treatise on Stones*, and *Moral Characters of Men*, and laid the foundations for anatomy and physiology.

c. 250 BC   HEROPHILUS, the first true anatomist, was one of the first Greek doctors to carry out dissections, discovered and named the prostate and duodenum.

25 BC The Greek physician AULUS CORNELIUS CELSUS was born. He wrote *De Medicina* and clearly described the presence and symptoms of calculi, urologic surgery, insertion of a catheter, and extraction of the stone with a lithotomy scoop.

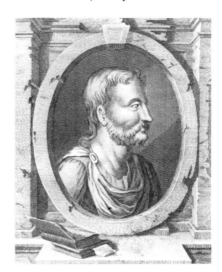

Aulus Cornelius Celsus
(25 BC–AD 50)

40 AD DIOSCORIDES born.
A Greek physician and pharmacologist who studied the medicinal properties of plants and minerals and described them in *De Materia Medica.*

129 AD GALEN was born in Pergamum, Asia Minor.
He noted the functions of the bladder and kidneys, and that flies were attracted to the urine of diabetics, thus denoting loss of sugar in such patients.

132 AD ARETAEUS OF CAPPADOCIA wrote *De causis et signis morborum,* and his description of the kidneys suggests that he was aware of the ducts of Bellini, but he considered the kidneys to be glands.

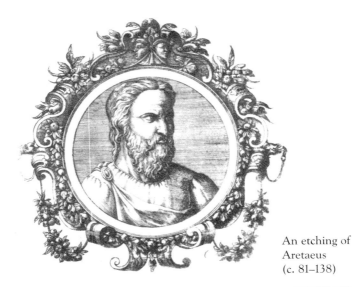

An etching of
Aretaeus
(c. 81–138)

625 AD PAUL OF AEGINA born.
Alexandrian physician and surgeon famed for his encyclopedia
Epitomae medicae libri septem, which contained descriptions of
lithotomy.

643 AD CHEN CHUAN born.
A Chinese physician who observed the symptoms of thirst and
production of sweet urine (diabetes).

850 AD RHAZES born.
Great Arab physician, ranked with HIPPOCRATES in his
portrayal of disease, who wrote *Liber de variolis el morbilis,* and
described stones, allergy and tuberculosis.

936 AD ALBUCASIS (Abu 'l-Quasim) born in El-Zahara near Cordoba.
The greatest Islamic surgeon of the Middle Ages. He wrote *Al-
Tasrif,* in which surgical procedures for bladder stones
were described.

c. 1000   AVICENNA (Ibn Cena) wrote a five-volume work about this period, *Canon of Medicine (Al-Qanum fil-Tibb)*. He recommended insertion of a louse into the urethral meatus of patients with urinary retention and this method was used for many centuries.

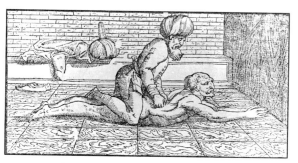

Avicenna (980–1037) massaging a man's back

1210   GUILIELMO SALICETTI born.
An Italian surgeon at Bologna who gave one of the earliest accounts of dropsy.

1307   JOHN OF ARDERNE born.
The first great English surgeon, noted for the revival of successful corrective surgery for ischiorectal abscess and fistula.

1340   Bile stones, or gallstones, were first observed by Italian physician, GENTILE DA FOLIGNO.

1458   HENNIG SEBASTIAN BRANDT born.
A German alchemist who discovered phosphorus in urine.

1478   GIROLAMO FRACASTORO born.
An Italian physician who proposed a possible cause for infectious diseases in *De contagionibus*, and introduced the term 'syphilis' in his work *Syphilidis sive de morbo Gallico*.

1500 CHU CHEN-HENG born.
An early Chinese endocrinologist who wrote on the use of urine extracts in infertility and dysmenorrhea.

1500 PIERRE FRANCO born.
A French surgeon who introduced the method of suprapubic cystotomy for the removal of stones, and published one of the first monographs on hernia.

1500 THIERRY DE HERY born.
A French physician who wrote a treatise on syphilis in which he recommended guaiacum from resin of the guaiacum tree, to be taken internally, or mercury for injection or fumigation.

1510 BARTOLOMMEO EUSTACHIO born.
A professor of anatomy in Rome who described the Eustachian tube, Eustachian valve in the fetus, thoracic duct, suprarenal bodies and abducent nerve. He wrote *Opuscula anatomica* (1564), which contained studies on the kidney.

1521 A description of appendix vermiformis, previously known as 'the worm of the bowel', or 'caecum intestinum', was made by Italian anatomist and surgeon JACOPO BERENGARIO DA CARPI. He also gave a clear description of the thymus, and performed a vaginal hysterectomy.

1527 French physician, JACQUES DE BETHENCOURT, described syphilis as morbus venereus.

1535 SANTO DE BARLETTA MARIANO born.
An Italian surgeon who described the perineal median operation for stone in the bladder.

1540 The term 'French gonorrhea' was first used by the Swiss physician, PARACELSUS, to denote syphilis, a terminology that created confusion between syphilis and gonorrhea for the next three centuries.

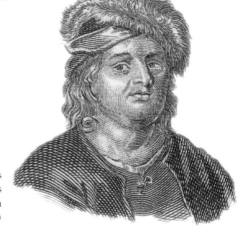

Paracelsus, also known as Theoprastus Bombastus von Hohenheim (1493–1541)

1542 The medicinal use of digitalis (foxglove) in dropsy and other conditions was described by Bavarian physician and botanist, LEONHART FUCHS.

1556 The suprapubic cystotomy procedure was first performed by French surgeon, PIERRE FRANCO.

1561 GABRIELE FALLOPPIO published his *Observaciones Anatomicae*. He differentiated the mucosa, submucosa and muscular coats of the viscera, described the valvulae conniventes of the small intestine and the sphincter at the end of the biliary apparatus, detailed the three muscular coats of the bladder and the internal sphincter, and the structure and functions of the kidney. He also propounded the idea that the renal papillae distilled urine from the blood.

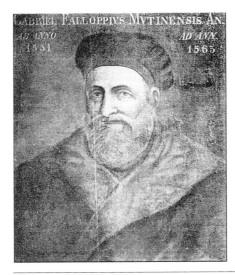

Gabriele Falloppio
(1523–1562)

1564 One of the earliest illustrations of the structure of the
kidneys, the thoracic duct, and the suprarenal glands was
given by BARTOLOMMEO EUSTACHIO, the celebrated Italian
physician from Rome.

1579 JAN BAPTISTA VAN HELMONT born.
A Dutch physician and founder of biochemistry who
described lipemia in diabetes mellitus.

1580 JEAN RIOLAN born.
An early French endocrinologist who described the
seminiferous tubules, and introduced the term 'capsulae
suprarenalis' for the adrenals.

1585 CASPAR BARTHOLIN, THE ELDER born.
A Danish physician who described a humor in the cavity
of adrenals, passed to the kidneys and then urine.

1588 The first treatise on diseases of the bladder, kidneys and
urethra was written by FRANCIS DIAZ, a Spanish surgeon and
the founder of modern urology.

1591 Italian physician, SEBASTIANUS PETRITIUS, recognized that the discharge from the penis in gonorrhea is pus, not semen.

1607 FRANCIS GLISSON born.
A surgeon from Britain who wrote *De Rachitide* and described the liver capsule with its blood supply and the bile duct sphincter.

1621 THOMAS WILLIS born.
A famous British anatomist who wrote on gout and diabetes. He advocated the use of colchicum for treatment of gout and as a prophylactic, also wrote on renal stones, and noted the effects of weather on joints of those with gout.

Thomas Willis
(1621–1675)

1628 ROBERT BOYLE born.
A British physician who proved that air was necessary for life and combustion, and wrote a book of remedies, including one for urinary calculi.

1628 MARCELLO MALPIGHI born.
The founder of microscopical anatomy from Bologna in Italy who described capillary anastomosis, discovered the uriniferous tubules (Malpighian bodies) and observed the ductus epoophori.

1641 REGNIER DE GRAAF born.
An eminent Dutch physician who was one of the first to experiment on the pancreas and published a treatise on pancreatic juice, described the Graafian follicle, and coined the term 'ovary'.

1642 *Liber de Rheumatismo et Pleuritide Dorsali*, a famous work on gout, rheumatic fever, acute polyarthritis, gouty arthritis, and rheumatoid arthritis, was published posthumously based on the writings of the French physician, GUILLAUME DE BAILLOU.

1643 LORENZO BELLINI born.
He described the gross anatomy of the kidney, discovered the renal excretory ducts (Bellini ducts) (1662), and explained fever.

1645 JEAN MERY born.
A surgeon from Paris who described the Cowper glands related to the male urethra, later named after WILLIAM COWPER who re-described them.

1651 FRÈRE JACQUES DE BEAULIEU born.
A French Franciscan lay brother and itinerant lithotomist. During his 19-year career, he is purported to have performed 4500 lithotomies and 2000 hernia operations.

1651 NATHANIEL HIGHMORE from Hampshire, England described the antrum of Highmore, and suggested that the suprarenals have an absorbent function of exudates from the large vessels. He wrote *Corporis Humani Disquisitio Anatomicae* and several other works.

1653 JOHANN CONRAD BRUNNER born.
A Swiss anatomist who conducted the first experiments on endocrinology, demonstrated the symptoms of thirst and polyuria of diabetes, and described the duodenal glands (Brunner glands).

1657 WILLIAM MUSGRAVE born.
An English physician who published a series of case studies on arthritis with urethral discharge, arthritis with psoriasis, and arthritis with renal colic.

1665 A classic description of the gross anatomy of the kidney was provided by one of the greatest medical thinkers of his time, LORENZO BELLINI of Florence, Italy, who discovered the renal excretory ducts (Bellini ducts), and explained fever.

1665 WILLIAM COWPER born.
An English surgeon who wrote *Myotomia Reformata* and *Anatomy of Human Bodies*, and described the pair of glands (Cowper glands) close to the male urethra.

1668 An early account on the structure of the testicles was given by Dutch physician, REGNIER DE GRAAF.

1670 THOMAS WILLIS noted the presence of sugar in the urine of diabetics.

1671 GEORGE CHEYNE born.
A Scottish physician and eminent writer who wrote *A New Theory of Fevers, An Essay on Method of Treating the Gout,* and *The English Malady or Treatise of Nervous Diseases.*

1681 GIOVANNI SANTORINI born.
An Italian anatomist who described the accessory duct
of the pancreas (Santorini duct) in *Observationes Anatomicae.*

1683 A classic treatise on gout, *Tractus de Podagra et de
Hydrope,* was written by THOMAS SYDENHAM, often known as
the 'English Hippocrates' due to his observation and
classic descriptions of diseases such as gout, dropsy and
chorea.

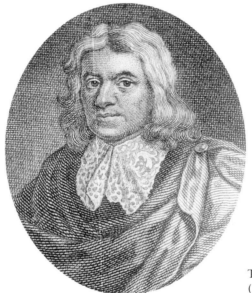

Thomas Sydenham
(1624–1689)

1688 WILLIAM CHESELDEN born.
A chief surgeon at St Thomas' Hospital, London, who
published a syllabus on human anatomy, and did
extensive studies in lithotomy.

1688 The symptoms of thirst and polyuria, indicative of diabetes,
were induced in dogs by surgical incision of their pancreas by
JOHANN CONRAD BRUNNER of Switzerland, who also described
the duodenal glands (Brunner glands).

1693   ANTOINE FERREIN born.
A surgeon and anatomist from Montpellier who described the cortical pyramids of the kidney and bile canaliculi, which are unconnected to the lobules.

1706   BENJAMIN FRANKLIN born.
An American scientist and statesman who suffered from and wrote on gout.

1708   *Institutiones Medicae in Usus Annuae Exercitationes Domesticos Gigestae* (including a description of gout) was written by Dutch chemist and physician, HERMANN BOERHAAVE, who also gave a classic description of urea.

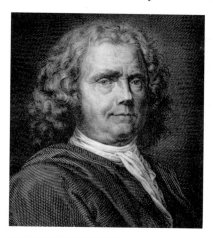

Hermann Boerhaave
(1668–1738)

1710   ALEXIS LITTRÉ of Paris proposed an artificial anus in the colon (colostomy), advising the opening of the sigmoid flexure in the iliac region in certain cases of imperforate anus.

1710   WILLIAM HEBERDEN THE ELDER born.
A London physician who described the association of renal stones with urinary tract infection.

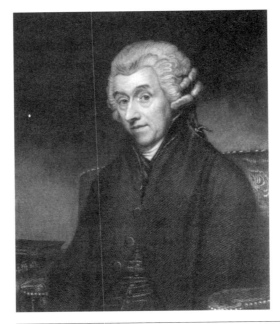

William Heberden
(1710–1801)

1713   MATTHEW DOBSON born.
A British physician and early endocrinologist who wrote
Experiments and Observations on the Urine in Diabetes, showed
the presence of sugar in urine and blood, and described
hyperglycemia.

1719   The Littré glands in the mucous membrane of the
spongy part of the urethra were described by ALEXIS LITTRÉ,
an anatomist and surgeon from Paris.

1727   Two feet of gangrenous bowel were resected from a
strangulated hernia for the first time (intestinal resection) by
KARL A RAMDOHR of Halle.

1729   WILLIAM BUCHAN born.
A Scottish physician who wrote three important works,
Domestic Medicine, Advice to Mothers and *Treatise on Venereal
Disease.*

1733 KASPAR FRIEDRICH WOLFF born.
A Berlin anatomist who described ren primordialis
(Wolffian body), ureter primordialis (Wolffian duct), and
proposed the theory of epigenesis.

1734 French physician, FRANÇOIS DE LA PEYRONIE, published
his review of ejaculatory dysfunction, and articles on
pathogenesis of penile fibrosis. Peyronie disease was first
described by VAN BUREN and KEYES in their treatise on
genitourinary disorders. The genetic factor was
recognized by WILMA BOAS and colleagues at the Johns
Hopkins Hospital in 1982.

1734 JOHANN GOTTLIEB WALTER born.
An anatomist in Berlin who gave his name to the
smallest branch of the splanchnic nerve passing through
the renal plexus (Walter nerve).

1742 CARL WILHELM SCHEELE born.
A Swedish urologist who
studied and analyzed urine
and made an examination of
pulverized bladder calculi
from patients with gouty
arthritis which led to the
discovery of uric acid and
calculus acid.

Carl Wilhelm Scheele
(1742–1786)

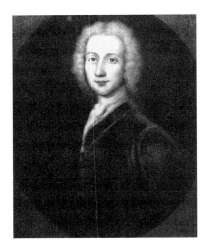

Robert Whytt
(1714–1766)

1742 ROBERT WHYTT published a paper on the possibility of
dissolving bladder stones with lime water and soap
injections, and wrote a small book on the subject in 1752.

1745 PETER JOHANN FRANK born.
A Bavarian physician who was the first to describe
diabetes insipidus (1794) and to differentiate it from
diabetes mellitus.

1749 BENJAMIN BELL born.
A surgeon at the Royal Edinburgh Infirmary who
differentiated between syphilis and gonorrhea in his
Gonorrhoea Virulenta and Lues Venera (1793).

1752 ANTONIO SCARPA born.
A Italian surgeon, anatomist, and ophthalmologist who wrote
Traité des Hernies, (1814), one of the first scientific
monographs on hernia.

1755 ANTOINE FRANÇOIS FOURCROY born.
A French chemist who gave an account of lumpy tissues
in a corpse which he named 'adipocere', and worked with
VANQUELIN in isolating urea.

1756 SIR EVERARD HOME born.
A surgeon at St George's Hospital who described the median lobe of the prostate (Home lobe) and published *Lectures on Comparative Anatomy, Practical Observations.*

1756 JOSEPH ADAMS born.
A British physician who wrote *Supposed Hereditary Properties of Disease*, and described gout, scrofula and goiter in cretinism.

1757 WILLIAM CHARLES WELLS born.
An English physician who demonstrated the presence of albumin and blood in the urine of patients with renal dropsy (1812).

1761 GIOVANNI BATTISTA MORGAGNI, the founder of pathological anatomy from Forli in Italy, discovered several anatomical structures which are named after him, noted syphilitic tumors of the brain, tuberculosis of the kidney, and wrote *Gout and other Pains of the Joints.*

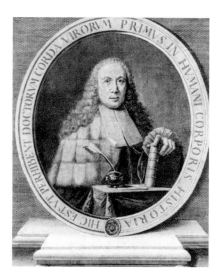

Giovanni Battista Morgagni
(1682–1771)

1765   JAMES WILSON born.
An English surgeon who described the muscle fibers derived from the levator ani surrounding the urethra, found above the triangular ligament (Wilson muscles).

1766   WILLIAM HYDE WOLLASTON born.
A British chemist who demonstrated the presence of uric acid, calcium, and ammonium in urinary stones (1797), and noted the occurrence of bladder stones in patients with cystinuria (1810).

1768   PHILIP SYNG PHYSICK born.
The father of American surgery who first performed a urethrotomy or internal longitudinal incision (1796) and successfully treated gouty arthritis and bladder stones.

1770   Cancer of the scrotum, the first occupational cancer (chimney sweep's cancer), was described by British surgeon, PERCIVALL POTT.

1770   The association between edema and coagulable substances in urine (nephrotic syndrome) was first observed by Italian anatomist, DOMENICO COTUGNO.

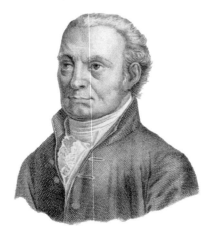

Domenico Cotugno
(1736–1822)

1775 CARL W SCHEELE of Sweden published his monograph *Chemical Treatise on Air and Fire*. He examined pulverized bladder calculi and isolated uric acid and calculus acid.

1776 The first surgeon to perform cecostomy, the opening of the cecum onto the right iliac region through a peritoneal incision in a patient with carcinoma of the rectum, was H PILLORE of Rouen.

1776 MATTHEW DOBSON, a British physician, published *Experiments and Observations on the Urine in Diabetes*, showed the presence of sugar in urine and the blood, and described hyperglycemia.

1780 The yeast test for detection of sugar in urine was devised by Edinburgh physician, FRANCIS HOME, who pioneered experimental inoculation against measles and published his research on croup, diabetes and other areas in *Medical Facts and Experiments*.

1785 Richter hernia, where only part of the lumen protrudes, was described by German surgeon, AUGUSTE GOTTLIEB RICHTER of Göttingen.

1785 English physician, WILLIAM WITHERING, established use of digitalis (foxglove) in the treatment of dropsy in his *An Account of the Foxglove*, and described the medicinal uses of the plant *Cicuta* in the treatment of cancer and syphilis.

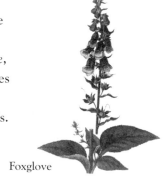

Foxglove

1786   An elevated papule in the penis or vulva in primary
        syphilis (Hunter chancre) was described by Scottish
        surgeon, JOHN HUNTER, and published in his *On Venereal
        Diseases*. A founder of surgical pathology, he described
        lymphogranuloma venereum, a sexually transmitted disease
        caused by *Chlamydia trachomatis*, and first attempted to
        separate syphilis from gonorrhea.

John Hunter
(1728–1793)

1786   JAMES O'BEIRNE born.
        An Irish surgeon who described the O'Beirne sphincter, a
        band at the junction of the colon and the rectum.

1788   Injury to the pancreas as a cause of diabetes was suggested by
        English physician, THOMAS CAWLEY.

1789   RICHARD BRIGHT born.
        A physician at Guy's Hospital, London who differentiated
        renal dropsy from cardiac dropsy and described chronic non-
        suppurative nephritis (Bright disease) in 1827.

1789   The suturing of a bladder after rupture was first suggested by
        BENJAMIN BELL, and first done by Willet of St Bartholomew's
        Hospital, London.

1789   EDWARD DONOVAN born.
        An Irish pharmacist who prepared and marketed
        Donovan solution, containing iodides of arsenic and
        mercury, for application to cutaneous and venereal sores.

1790   Urological surgery was introduced as a specialty by
        PIERRE J DESAULT and FRANÇOIS CHOPART of Paris, who also
        published treatises on venereal disease and on stones in the
        bladder and kidneys.

1790   JACQUES LISFRANC born.
        A French surgeon who advocated the extirpation of the
        rectum as treatment for cancer.

1792   GASTON SÈGALAS born.
        A French urologist and pioneer in endoscopy in urology, who
        improved the method initially described by PHILLIP BOZZONI.

1793   An operation for strangulated femoral hernia was described
        by ANTONIO DE GIMBERNAT, a surgeon from Barcelona in
        Spain.

1793 CHARLES ASTON KEY born.
A British surgeon who performed successful ligations for aneurysms, and described a surgical method for relieving strangulated inguinal hernia.

1793 Descriptions and engravings produced by Scottish surgeon, MATTHEW BAILLIE, included cancer of the stomach, bladder, esophagus and testes, and are generally regarded as reaching new heights of clarity.

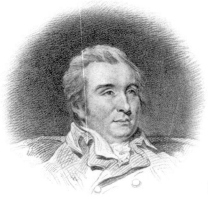

Matthew Baillie
(1761–1823)

1793 THOMAS ADDISON born.
A physician at Guy's Hospital, London who described a disorder resulting from destruction of the renal glands (Addison disease).

1794 The first description of diabetes insipidus was given by PETER JOHANN FRANK of Bavaria, who also differentiated it from other forms of diabetes.

1795 Urethrotomy, or internal longitudinal incision, was first performed by American surgeon, PHILIP SYNG PHYSICK of Philadelphia, who also successfully treated gouty arthritis and bladder stones.

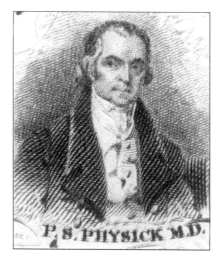

Philip Syng Physick
(1768–1837)

1795   ALFRED VELPEAU born.
A surgeon in Paris who has several anatomical structures
named after him, including the inguinal canal, ischiorectal
fossa, and tela subserosa around the kidney.

1796   JEAN BAPTISTE BOUILLAUD born.
A French physician who correlated carditis with acute
rheumatic fever (Bouillaud syndrome).

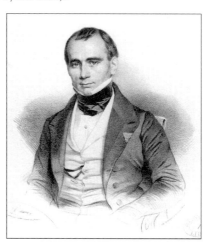

Jean Baptiste Bouillaud
(1796–1881)

1797 WILLIAM HYDE WOLLASTON, a British chemist, demonstrated the presence of various substances, including uric acid, calcium and ammonium in urinary stones, and noted the occurrence of bladder stones in patients with cystinuria.

1799 PHILLIPE RICORD born.
An American pioneer in venereology who demonstrated the different etiology of syphilis and gonorrhea, and described the three stages of syphilis.

1803 JEAN GASPARD BLAISE GOYRAND born.
A French surgeon who described a type of inguinal hernia which protruded into a partial sac.

1803 JUSTUS VON LIEBIG born.
A German chemist who discovered chloroform, studied nutrition and the degradation of proteins to purines, and urea and uric acid.

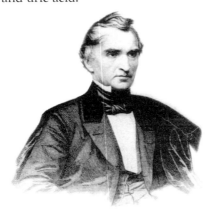

Justus von Liebig
(1803–1873)

1804 PHILLIP BOZZINI invented a cystoscope for the bladder, and in 1879 MAX NITZE, a German urologist, developed a lens system for it.

1804   JOSEPH DIETL born.
A Polish physician who described recurrent pain in the costavertebral angle with vomiting, nausea, tachycardia and hypotension due to ureteral obstruction (Dietl crisis).

1805   SAMUEL DAVID GROSS born.
An American surgeon who introduced laparotomy for ruptured bladder, suprapubic incision for the prostate, distinguished prostatic hypertrophy from bladder disease, and wrote *Elements of Pathological Anatomy*.

1806   APPOLLINAIRE BOUCHARDAT born.
A French chemist who used polariscopic and chemical methods to detect diabetes, developed diets, and invented gluten-free bread.

1806   Prostatism was treated transurethrally via perineal urethrotomy by SIR WILLIAM BLIZARD of London.

1809   JOHN STOUGH BOBB born.
An American surgeon who described cholecystotomy for removal of gallstones.

1809   FRIEDRICH GUSTAVE JACOB HENLE born.
A German anatomist who discovered the external sphincter of the bladder, the looped portion of the uriniferous tubule (loop of Henle), and described the columnar and ciliated epithelial cells.

1810   WILLIAM CHARLES WELLS, an American physician, detected albumin in urine in cases of anascara, 30 years before BRIGHT, and observed hematuria and albuminuria in cases of scarlet fever and dropsy.

1810 The amino acid, cystine, was isolated from urinary calculi by an English physician and chemist, WILLIAM HYDE MACARTHUR.

1810 HENRY SAVAGE born.
A gynecologist at the Samaritan Hospital in London who described the perineal body between the anus and the vulva (Savage perineal body).

1811 THOMAS BLIZARD CURLING born.
A London surgeon who discovered acute duodenal ulceration (Curling ulcer), and published *Diseases of the Testis* and *Diseases of the Rectum*.

1812 CHARLES P J DISAY born.
An American physician who dedicated his life to the study of syphilis and made important contributions to the famous venereal clinic in St Louis with JEAN ALFRED FOURNIER.

1812 Perforated appendix was recognized as a cause of death by London physician, JAMES PARKINSON.

1813 GEORGE OWEN REES born.
An English physician who devised the Rees test, used for the detection of albumin in urine, using tannic acid in alcoholic solution.

1813 QUINTON GIBBON born.
An American surgeon who described a large inguinal hernia with hydocele (Gibbon hernia).

1813 JOHN BLACKALL, one of the first physicians to demonstrate albuminuria in dropsy, published his findings in *Observations on the Nature and Cure of Dropsies*.

1813 JOHAN FLORENZE HELLER born.
An Austrian physician who devised the nitric acid test for detecting protein in urine, and wrote an important work on urinary calculi (1860).

1814 GOLDING BIRD born.
A British urologist who wrote a monograph on urinary deposits, described oxaluria, and wrote *Elements of Natural Philosophy*.

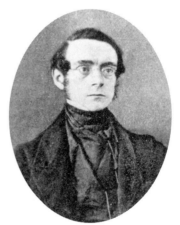

Golding Bird
(1814–1854)

1814 One of the first scientific monographs on hernia, *Traité des Hernies*, was written by Italian anatomist ANTONIO SCARPA.

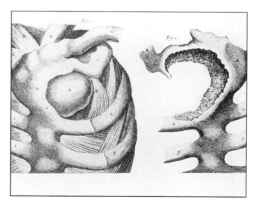

A page from one of Scarpa's books

1814 HENRY BENCE JONES born.
An English physician who pioneered chemical and microscopical examination of urine prior to diagnosing diabetes. He also wrote on renal calculi, gout, and has numerous eponyms: Bence Jones albumin, cylinders, myeloma, proteins and reaction.

1814 Colchicine was extracted from the meadow saffron, and was the only real treatment for gout until the development of anti-inflammatory agents.

1815 MICHEL EUGÈNE CHEVREUL, a French chemist, showed that the sugar in diabetic urine was glucose.

1815 JAMES ARCHIBALD JACQUES born.
He invented the first soft urethral catheter (Jacques catheter) while production manager of a London rubber mill.

1816 SIR WILLIAM BOWMAN born.
An English anatomist who developed the concept of glomerular filtration and tubular secretion (1842), and described the capsules in the kidneys that filter blood (Bowman capsule).

1816 LUDWIG MORITZ HIRSCHFELD born.
A Polish anatomist who described the lingual branch of the facial nerve (Hirschfeld nerve), and the posterior renal sympathetic ganglion.

1817 JOHANN B V L CHIARI born.
An Austrian gynecologist who discovered the Chiari–Frommel syndrome consisting of postpartum galactorrhea with pituitary adenoma (and atrophy of the uterus).

1817   EDOUARD BROWN-SÉQUARD born.
A French neurophysiologist who demonstrated the importance of the suprarenal capsule, and described hemiplegia associated with anesthesia (Brown-Séquard syndrome).

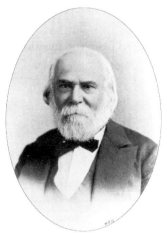

Edouard Brown-Séquard
(1817–1894)

1817   ALPHONSE F M GUÉRIN born.
A surgeon at the Hôtel Dieu, Paris who described the terminal portion of the male urethra.

1818   Urethritis, conjunctivitis, and arthritis were first described by BENJAMIN COLLINS BRODIE of St George's Hospital, London.

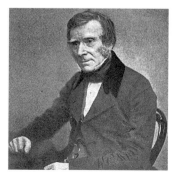

Benjamin Collins Brodie
(1783–1862)

1818   EDME JOULES MAUMENÉ born.
A French chemist who devised the Maumené test to detect sugar in urine by adding stannous chloride to give a distinct brown color.

1819   A procedure for opening an obstructed bowel above the site of obstruction and allowing the contents to escape (enterotomy) was first suggested by MANNOURY.

1819   WENZEL TREITZ born.
A pathological anatomist at Prague who described retroperitoneal hernia through the duodenojejunal recess (Treitz hernia), and the suspensory ligament of the duodenum (Treitz ligament).

1820   SIR HENRY THOMPSON born.
An English genitourinary surgeon who described the surgical treatment of urinary bladder tumors and wrote extensively on urethral stricture, and *Enlarged Prostate, Its Pathology and Treatment.*

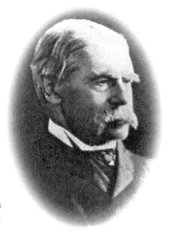

Sir Henry Thompson
(1820–1904)

1820 The amino acid, glycine, was isolated from a hydrosylate of gelatin by HENRI BRACONNET, who named it 'sugar of gelatin'.

1820 JOSEPH GERLACH born.
An anatomist at Erlangen who described the lymphatic follicles in the mucous membrane of the Eustachian tube, and the mucosal fold near the orifice of the appendix (Gerlach valve).

1821 The accumulation of urea in the blood after extirpation of the kidneys was observed by JOHN B A DUMAS and Swiss physician, JEAN LOUIS PREVOST.

1822 The method of bruising a urinary stone with surgical instruments (lithotrity) was first practiced by M LEROY ETIOLLES.

1823 TRUMANN HOFFMAN SQUIRE born.
An American surgeon who wrote a treatise on stricture of the urethra and designed a catheter.

1824 SIR SAMUEL WILKS born.
An English physician who gave a definite account of myasthenia gravis (Wilks syndrome), the relationship between renal conditions and nephritic syndrome, the causes of pyemia, and an account of alcoholic paraplegia.

1824 JEAN CIVIALE invented a lithotrite.

1825 FESSENDEN NOTT OTIS born.
An American urologist who designed a method for internal urethrotomy and introduced the use of local anesthesia in urology (1884).

1825   NATHAN BOZEMANN born.
An American surgeon who designed a double-channeled
urethral catheter (Bozemann catheter).

1825   JEAN MARTIN CHARCOT born.
An eminent French neurologist who contributed vastly to this
field, and also carried out work on biliary passages, the liver,
and kidneys.

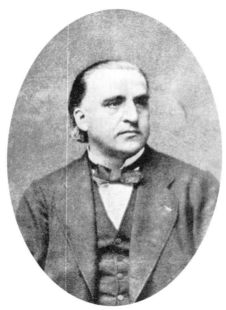

Jean Martin Charcot
(1825–1893)

1826   ALPHONSE DUMONTPALLIER born.
He devised the Dumontpallier test for detection of bile
pigments using iodine.

1826   EDMÉ FELIX ALFRED VULPIAN born.
A physician from Paris, who demonstrated the presence of an
active vital substance in the adrenal glands, later named
epinephrine.

1827   JULIUS NESSLER born.
A German chemist from Karlsruhe who prepared
Nessler reagent, a test for ammonia, used in the analysis
of blood, urea and plasma proteins.

1827   The term hyperemia was introduced by French
physician, GABRIEL ANDRAL.

1827   A classic description of chronic non-suppurative nephritis
(Bright disease) was given by RICHARD BRIGHT of Guy's
Hospital, London, one of the earliest to focus on renal
disease. He differentiated renal dropsy from cardiac dropsy
and described hiatus hernia (1836) and wrote *Account of a
Remarkable Misplacement of the Stomach.*

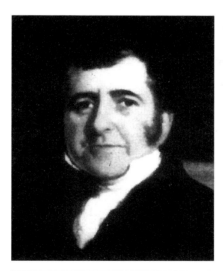

Richard Bright
(1789–1858)

1829   Urea was synthesized from potassium cyanate and
ammonium sulfate by German chemist, FRIEDRICH WÖHLER,
who specialized in gynecology, this signaled the founding of
organic chemistry.

1829 FREDERICK WILLIAM PAVY born.
An English biochemist who studied carbohydrate metabolism and diabetes. He correlated hyperglycemia and glycosuria, described cyclic or recurrent albuminuria (Pavy disease), and the involvement of the joints in typhoid.

1829 JOHN L W THUDICHUM born.
A German physician in London who pioneered studies of phospholipids and devised the Thudichum test, to detect creatinine using ferric chloride as reagent.

1829 GEORGE HARLEY born.
A Scottish physician who studied intermittent hematuria, later known as paroxysmal nocturnal hematuria (Harley disease).

1830 HENRI FERDINAND DOLBEAU born.
A Paris surgeon who described the Dolbeau operation for lithotomy, in which the stone is crushed in the bladder through a median incision in the urethra.

1830 A modern monograph on the structure and diseases of the testicles was published by SIR ASTLEY PASTON COOPER of Guy's Hospital in London.

1830 SIR WILLIAM ROBERTS born.
An English physician who devised the Roberts test for the detection of albumin in urine, with a solution of magnesium sulfate and sulfuric acid.

1831 Lithotrity was introduced into America by JACOB RANDOLPH of Philadelphia, MOTT of New York, WARREN of Boston, and SMITH of Baltimore followed close behind.

1832   LÉON LABBÉ born.
A Paris surgeon who developed pre-anesthetic medication, and gave his name to the Labbé triangle between the inferior border of the liver and lower border of the 9th costal cartilage.

1832   NICOLAUS RUDINGER born.
A professor of anatomy at Munich who described the muscles internal to the circular fibers of the rectum (Rudinger muscle).

1832   JEAN A FOURNIER born.
A Paris professor who made several important contributions to the study of syphilis, and gave his name to fulminating gangrene of the scrotum and perineum in diabetic patients.

1833   EDUARD VON WAHL born.
A German surgeon who described distention of the proximal portion of obstructed bowel (Wahl sign), and the systolic murmur over an injured artery.

1834   HUGO SCHIFF born.
A German chemist who worked in Florence, Italy, where he devised the Schiff test to detect carbohydrates in urine, with sulfuric acid, glacial acetic acid and alcohol as reagents.

1835   THOMAS GEORGE MORTON born.
An American surgeon from Philadelphia who carried out the successful removal of an inflamed appendix and gave a complete description of metatarsalgia (Morton disease).

1835   Irish surgeon, ABRAHAM COLLES, wrote a treatise on syphilis, *Practical Observation on the Venereal Disease*, in which he referred to immunity acquired to syphilis by a healthy mother in bearing a syphilitic child (Colles law). In his *Surgical Anatomy* he described Colles fascia, the fascia in which urine extravasates after rupture of the bulbous urethra.

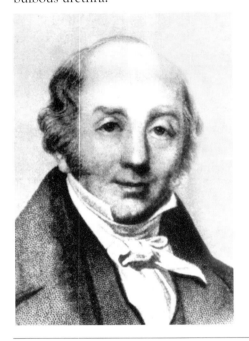

Abraham Colles
(1773–1843)

1835   CLAES G W NYLANDER born.
A Swedish chemist who detected dextrose in the urine (Nylander test).

1836   A parasitic flagellated protozoan (*Trichomonas vaginalis*), found in the vagina and male urinary tract, was first recognized by ALFRED DONNÉ of Paris.

1836   AUSTIN FLINT JUNIOR born.
        An American physiologist after whom the vascular arches
        at the bases of the pyramids of the kidneys (Flint arcade)
        are named.

1836   WILHELM EBSTEIN born.
        A German physician at Göttingen who described the
        congenital displacement of the tricuspid valve into the right
        ventricle (Ebstein anomaly), and the hyaline degeneration of
        the epithelial cells in the renal tubules.

1837   ANDRÉ VICTOR CORNIL born.
        A French urologist who wrote on the pathology of the
        kidneys, and showed sodium urate in joints in gout.

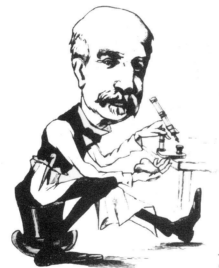

André Victor Cornil
(1837–1908)

1838   The occurrence of albuminuria in fevers (febrile albuminuria)
        was described by MARTIN SOLON of Paris.

1838   RICHARD DAVY born.
A London surgeon who gave his name to a wooden sound
for insertion into the rectum to stop bleeding in the iliac
artery (Davy lever).

1838   The reduced excretion of urea and solids in the urine,
anazoturia, was named by R WILLIS.

1839   The Amussat operation, a lumbar colotomy for obstruction
of the colon, was performed by JEAN ZULLEMA AMUSSAT in
Paris, France.

1839   BERNARD NAUNYN born.
A professor of clinical medicine in Bern, Switzerland who
devoted his career to metabolism in diabetes (1898) and
diseases of the liver and pancreas, described acidosis (1906),
and founded the *Archiv für Experimentale Pathologie und
Pharmakologie.*

1840   The procedure for enterotomy was first performed in Paris by
AUGUSTE NÉLATON, a French surgeon who used a rubber
urethral catheter, and also introduced electrocautery into
surgery.

1840   JOSEPH CASIMIR GRYNFELTT born.
A French gynecologist from Montpellier who described the
superior lumbar triangle through which lumbar hernia occur
(Grynfeltt triangle).

1840   EDWARD WILHELM WELANDER born.
A physician from Stockholm, Sweden who described
chancroid or chancre found in the vulva but of nonvenereal
etiology (Welander ulcer).

1840   Intoxication due to poor kidney functioning (uremia) was described by French physician, PIERRE-ADOLPHE PIORRY.

1841   GEORGE OLIVER born.
An English pioneer in endocrinology who demonstrated the effect of injecting extracts of the suprarenal gland, producing contraction of the arteries and accelerated heart rate, thereby increasing blood pressure.

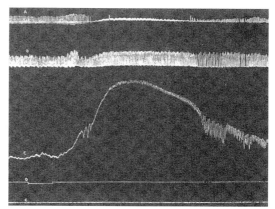

Chart of changes in blood pressure

1841   The Trommer test which detects dextrose in urine, using sodium hydroxide and copper sulfate as reagents, was devised by German chemist, KARL AUGUST TROMMER.

1841   Pyelonephritis, inflammation of the kidney, was described in pregnant women by PIERRE FRANÇOIS OLIVE RAYER of Paris.

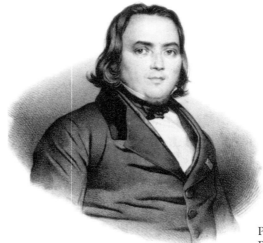

Pierre François Olive
Rayer (1793–1867)

1841 MAX JAFFE born.
A biochemist from Königsberg who introduced techniques for
detection of urobilin in urine and in the intestines, detection
of creatinine, and the isolation of indican in urine.

1842 CARL GUSSENBAUER born.
A German surgeon who devised an internal metal splint
(Gussenbauer clamp) for ununited fracture, and gave a
description of the first removal of a tumor in the bladder.

1842 VINCENZ CZERNY born.
A surgeon at Heidelberg who successfully resected
the esophagus in a human, removed a cancer of the large
bowel, and introduced the vaginal operation for carcinoma
of the uterus.

1842 CHARLES HENRY RALFE born.
A physician at the London Hospital who devised the Ralfe test for detection of acetone in urine, by adding hydroxide and iodide of potassium, and wrote *Urine* and *Diseases of the Kidney.*

1842 The idea that urine formation consisted of glomerular filtration and tubular secretion was proposed by the English physician, WILLIAM BOWMAN. He discovered the capsules in the kidneys that filter blood, and the Bowman membrane which separates the corneal epithelium from the substantia propria.

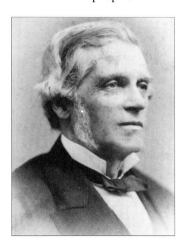

William Bowman
(1816–1892)

1842 ROBERT ULTZMANN born.
A German urologist who devised the Ultzmann test which detects bile pigments in urine, using potassium hydroxide as reagent.

1842 Severe dilatation of the upper urinary tract during pregnancy (hydronephrosis) was first shown at postmortem by JEAN CRUVEILHIER, professor of pathological anatomy at Paris.

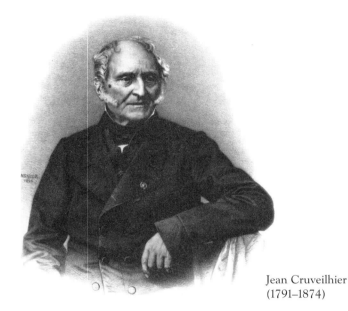

Jean Cruveilhier
(1791–1874)

1842   WILLIAM ANDERSON born.
A British urologist who described Anderson–Fabry disease
(1898), relating to a burning sensation in the hands and feet,
dark nodular skin lesions, and renal failure.

1843   CHARLES MEYMOTT TIDY born.
An English physician who devised the Tidy test which
detects albumin in the urine, using phenol and glacial
acetic acid as reagents.

1843   LUDWIG GEORG COURVOISIER born.
A surgeon in Switzerland and one of the first to remove
stones from the common bile duct. He formulated
Courvoisier law, relating to obstructive jaundice due to
gallstones in the common duct.

1843 The presence of albumin in the urine (albuminuria) of mothers with puerperal convulsions was observed by JOHN CHARLES LEVER, lecturer in midwifery at Guy's Hospital in London.

1843 A cylindrical structure of microscopic size (urinary cast) was observed in urine by SIMON of Vienna and HERMANN NASSE of Germany.

1843 EDMUND DRECHSEL born.
A Swiss chemist who devised the Drechsel test for bile, using phosphoric acid and sugar cane as reagents.

1843 REGINALD HEBER FITZ born.
An American pathologist who described the symptoms and signs of inflammation of the vermiform appendix, and named the condition appendicitis.

1843 The concept that urine formation in the kidneys was a simple process of filtration brought about by the hydrostatic pressure of the blood was proposed by CARL F W LUDWIG of Zurich, Switzerland.

1844 LEOPOLD SALKOWSKI born.
A Berlin chemist who described pentosuria, and devised tests for purine bases, cholesterol, creatinine, bile pigments, carbon monoxide in blood, glucose in urine, and hematoporphyrin.

1844 LUDWIG BREMER born.
An American physician who used methylene and eosin as reagents in his test for detecting sugar in the blood (Bremer test).

1844 HEINRICH FRITSCH born.
A German gynecologist who designed a double-channeled
uterine catheter (Fritsch catheter).

1844 FRIEDRICH GUSTAVE JACOB HENLE, the celebrated German
anatomist, was the first to demonstrate that urinary casts
originated in the kidney.

1844 EMMANUEL AUFRECHT born.
A German physician who first observed the association of
liver pathology with changes in the kidney in cases of
infectious jaundice (hepatorenal syndrome).

1845 An account of spermatic cord tumors (testicular tumor) was
given by French surgeon, EDME LÈSAUVAGE.

1846 THOMAS PRIDGIN TEALE of Leeds wrote one of the first
monographs on abdominal hernia, describing the protrusion
of a structure through an opening in the abdomen.

1846 ARTHUR FERGUSON McGILL born.
An English surgeon who performed the first suprapubic
prostatectomy.

1847 PAUL LANGERHANS born.
A German pathologist from Berlin who discovered the islets in
the pancreas which produce insulin (islets of Langerhans, 1869),
and insulinoma (Langerhans adenoma).

1847 English physician, HENRY BENCE JONES, described the
presence of albuminoid protein in the urine of a
patient with two fractured ribs, later named Bence Jones
proteinuria.

1851 FRANK THOMAS PAUL born.
A a physician at Guy's Hospital, London who employed the Paul tube to temporarily drain fecal matter after colostomy in cases of obstruction of the large bowel.

1851 FERDINAND C VALENTINE born.
A New York surgeon who described the patient supine at the edge of the operating table with legs hanging down, used for irrigating the urethra (Valentine position).

1851 THEODOR WEYLE born.
A chemist from France who devised the Weyle test, which detects creatinine using sodium nitroprusside as reagent.

1851 PAUL KRASKE born.
A surgeon from Freiburg who described an operation (Kraske operation) for carcinoma of the rectum, where the surgical approach is gained by excision of the sacrum and coccyx.

1852 JULIUS MULLER removed a cystine stone from the bladder of a young boy.

1852 MORITZ HOLL born.
A physician from Vienna who described the intercrural ligament found in front of the urinary meatus of the female.

1852 ACHILLE ETIENNE MALECOT born.
A French surgeon who designed a large-bore suprapubic urinary catheter (Malecot catheter).

1852   HENRY EALES born.
An English physician who wrote a review of the
appearance of the retina in patients with renal disease,
and on recurrent retinal and vitreous hemorrhage
(Eales disease).

1853   ROBERT TIGERSTEDT born.
A physiologist from Finland who discovered pressor
substance, formed in the kidneys (renin) and discharged
into the circulation of the renal glands, and carried out
studies on nerve response to mechanical stimulation.

1853   ALEXANDER HUGH FERGUSON born.
A Chicago surgeon who specialized in the treatment of hernia
and described a radical cure for femoral hernia.

1853   JAMES RUTHERFORD MORISON born.
A surgeon working in Newcastle, England who pioneered
pelvic surgery for women, published *Abdominal and Pelvic
Surgery* and also pioneered
surgical treatment for gallstones and gastric cancer.

1853   GEORGE MICHAEL EDEBOHLS born.
An American surgeon who introduced decortication to treat
chronic nephritis and later performed nephropexy in a
movable kidney with chronic nephritis.

1853   PAUL JULIUS POIRIER born.
A French surgeon who described the lymphatic gland
situated on the uterine artery where it crosses the urethra
(Poirier gland).

1853 KAREL MAYDL born.
A surgeon at Prague and Vienna who performed the first successful colostomy, and uretero-intestinal anastomosis, with insertion of the extroverted bladder into the rectum for ectopic vesicae.

1853 The fungus responsible for candidosis was named *Oidium albicans* by CHARLES P ROBIN.

1854 Acute or chronic fungal infection, generally seen in males and affecting the groin, perineum and perineal area (tinea cruris), was described by FRIEDRICH VON BÄRENSPRUNG.

1854 JAMES BROWN born.
A surgeon working at Johns Hopkins Hospital in Baltimore who catheterized male urethras.

1855 RUDOLPH VON JAKSCH born.
A physician in Prague who described pseudoleukemia, or acute hemolytic anemia in children (von Jaksch anemia), and was one of the first to investigate the presence of acetone bodies in the urine.

1855 ANATOLE M E CHAUFFARD born.
A French physician who gave his name to the point of tenderness below the right clavicle in cases of cholecystitis.

1855 ALBERT L S NEISSER born.
A German bacteriologist who discovered the gonorrhea bacterium (*Neisseria gonorrhoeae*) and succeeded OSCAR SIMON as professor of skin and venereal diseases at the University of Breslau.

1856 Arterial hypertension was recognized as the linking factor between renal disease and hypertension by German pathologist, LUDWIG TRAUBE.

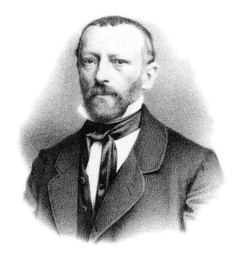

Ludwig Traube
(1818–1876)

1856 The occurrence of an active vital substance in the adrenal medulla was demonstrated by EDMÉ FELIX ALFRED Vulpian of Paris.

1857 Uremic pericarditis, which occurs in cases of renal failure, was studied by HEINRICH VON BAMBERGER of Germany.

1857 JOHN ALEXANDER MACWILLIAM born.
A physiologist at Aberdeen, Scotland, who gave the first account of death due to ventricular fibrillation, and devised the MacWilliam test for albuminuria.

1857 JAMES PERCIVAL TUTTLE born.
A New York surgeon who designed a rectal speculum with an electric light attached to its extremity, and capable of inflating the rectal ampulla (Tuttle proctoscope).

1857   The Scottish surgeon SIR WILLIAM FERGUSSON published *System of Practical Surgery.* He excelled in lithotomy, preferring to crush the stone *in situ*, and devised his own lithotrite for this purpose.

1857   Acetone in urine in cases of diabetes was shown by Prague physician, WILHELM PETTERS.

1857   JOHN BENJAMIN MURPHY born.
An American pioneer in vascular surgery who designed the Murphy button for intestinal anastomosis, and introduced the Murphy saline drip.

1857   SIR ARCHIBALD EDWARD GARROD born.
A London physician and a pioneer in the study of inborn errors of metabolism, including alkaptonuria, cystinuria and pentosuria (1909).

1858   WILLARD MYSON ALLEN born.
A Berlin physician who devised the Cornet forceps for holding litmus paper while testing urine.

1858   CARL HARKO VON NOORDEN born.
A Viennese physician who studied diabetes and laid down the principles of the antidiabetic diet before the insulin era.

1858   ISMAR ISIDOR BOAS born.
A German gastroenterologist who described hyperaesthesia below the right scapula posteriorly, and the 9th and 11th ribs, in acute cholecystitis (Boas sign).

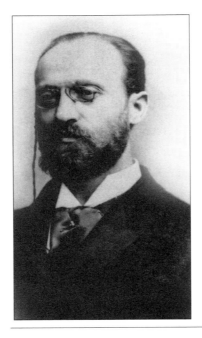

Ismar Isidor Boas
(1858–1942)

1858 OSKAR MINKOWSKI born.
A Lithuanian professor of medicine in Breslau who
established the role of the pancreas in diabetes, and showed
pituitary enlargement in acromegaly.

1859 MARK ARMAND RUFFIER born.
A pioneer in paleopathology who studied conditions such as
tuberculosis, arteriosclerosis and gallstones.

1859 JULIUS VON HOCHENEGG born.
A surgeon from Vienna who described an operation
for the removal of a malignant rectum through the
sacral route.

1860 GEORGE NEIL STEWART born.
A physician from Edinburgh who used (with JULIUS MOSES
ROGOFF) adrenocortical extract for the treatment
of adrenal insufficiency.

1860 Enucleation of the enlarged lateral lobes of the prostate through an external incision was carried out by Austrian surgeon, LEOPOLD RITTER VON DITTEL, one of the first specialists in urology.

1860 SIR WILLIAM WITHEY GULL born.
A physician at Guy's Hospital, London who described Gull disease or myxedema, and gave a clear description of arteriosclerotic atrophy of the kidney.

1860 A complete transposition in the abdomen and chest in a woman of 85 years, who was previously well, was described at postmortem by EDWARD PARKER YOUNG of England.

1860 The Hospital for Stone in London was opened. In 1946 St Peter's Hospital and the neighboring urological hospital, St Paul's, united and the Institute of Urology was established. In 1956, a trust for a lectureship in urology was founded, and the first lecture, 'Metabolic Causes of Renal Stone Formation', was given in 1958 by C E DENT.

1860 JOAQUIN DOMINGUEZ ALBARRÁN born.
A Cuban-born professor of medicine in France, who described the Albarrán gland in the prostate, Albarrán operation for nephropexy, and Albarrán test for kidney function.

1860 CHARLES ÉMILE ACHARD born.
A Paris physician who introduced a test for renal function, coined the term paratyphoid fever, and wrote on edema in Bright disease.

1861   The first experiments on dialysis were carried out by
THOMAS GRAHAM, a chemist from Glasgow, who used a
simple dialyzer made of parchment tied to the end of a large-
mouthed funnel.

1861   The association between gallstones and cancer was suggested
by FRIEDRICH THEODOR VON FRERICHS of Aurich in
Germany, in *Clinical Treatise on Diseases
of the Liver*.

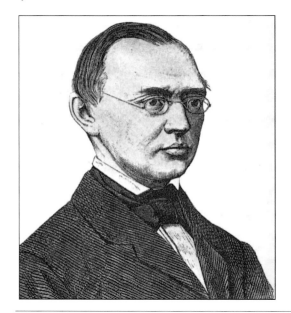

Friedrich Theodor
von Frerichs
(1819–1885)

1861   ERASTUS BRADLEY WOLCOT, American surgeon from
Benton, New York, was the first to perform nephrectomy.

1861   FRED NEUFELD born.
A German bacteriologist who described bacteriotropins and
demonstrated lysis of pneumococci by bile salts.

1861 FRIEDRICH OBERMAYER born.
An Austrian physiological chemist who devised the
Obermayer test which detects indican in urine, using lead
acetate as reagent.

1861 GEORGE E BREWER born.
An American surgeon who described Brewer kidney,
relating to hematogenous abscesses following septicemia,
and pyramidal reddened areas in the kidney, seen in
acute unilateral hematogenous pyelonephritis
(Brewer infarcts).

1861 HUGO VON FELEKI born.
A Hungarian urologist who devised an instrument for
massaging the prostate gland (Feleki instrument).

1862 MALCOLM LA SALLE HARRIS born.
A Chicago surgeon who described the hepatoduodenal
band, consisting of a fold of peritoneum from the gall
bladder to the cystic duct across the transverse colon
(Harris band).

1862 LOTHAR VON FRANKEL-HOCHWART born.
An Austrian neurologist who described cochlea,
vestibular and trigeminal lesions (Frankel-Hochwart disease)
seen in early syphilis.

1863 THOMAS JAMES WATKINS born.
A Chicago gynecologist who designed the Watkins operation,
for prolapse of the uterus where the bladder is separated from
the wall of the uterus, so that the uterus is left in position to
support the entire bladder.

1864 The Contagious Diseases Act, designed to combat the spread of venereal diseases, was passed in England.

1865 A condition where iron is deposited in the liver, skin and other organs leading to pigmentation, cirrhosis and diabetes (bronze diabetes) was first described by French physician, ARMAND TROUSSEAU.

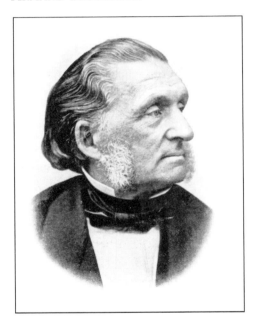

Armand Trousseau
(1801–1867)

1865 ADOLF SCHMIDT born.
A physician from Halle, Germany who devised the Schmidt test for detection of bilirubin in feces, with mercuric chloride as reagent.

1866 ARTHUR CUSHNY born.
A British pharmacologist at University College, London who described auricular fibrillation, and analyzed the process of urinary secretion which he recorded in *The Secretion of Urine*.

1866   FRIEDRICH G J HENLE published the first volume in his illustrated *Handbook of Systematic Anatomy*. A German anatomist who discovered the external sphincter of the bladder, the tubules of the kidney, and the medullary portion of the nephron between the proximal and distal tubules of the collecting system of the kidney, and the loop of Henle. Henle also demonstrated the importance of urinary casts in renal disease.

1867   MAX WILMS born.
        A German surgeon who studied a kidney tumor which bears his name (1899).

1868   JABEZ NORTH JACKSON born.
        An anatomist in Kansas who described the peritoneal attachment of the cecum, and the ascending colon to the right abdominal wall (Jackson membrane) producing obstruction of the bowel.

1868   WALTER BERNARD COFFEY born.
        A San Francisco surgeon who treated cancer by injecting an extract from the suprarenal cortex of the sheep.

1868   GUY L R HUNNER born.
        An American surgeon and gynecologist, and one of the first students at the Johns Hopkins Hospital, who described the Hunner ulcer (a chronic vesicle ulcer at the vertex of the bladder).

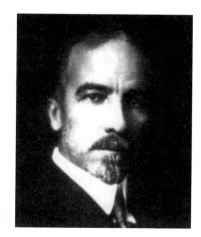

Guy L R Hunner (1868–1957)

1869   NICHOLAS CONSTANTIN PAULESCO born.
A Rumanian physician and pioneer in the study of diabetes who pointed out the causal relationship between diabetes and lesions of the pancreas.

1869   German surgeon, GUSTAV SIMON, demonstrated that a diseased kidney in a human patient could be surgically removed without detriment to the patient, providing that the remaining kidney was healthy.

1869   A form of arthritis of the hands and fingers in patients with rheumatic fever (Jaccoud disease) was described by French pathologist at Paris, SIGISMOND JACCOUD.

1869   ARTHUR BIEDL born.
A German physician who worked on neural control of the viscera through splanchnic centers, and also demonstrated the importance of adrenal glands in internal secretions.

1869   WILHELM SCHLESINGER born.
A Viennese physician who devised the Schlesinger test for detecting urobilin in the urine, using Lugol iodine.

1870   MANFRED BIAL born.
A German physician who devised the Bial test for detecting pentose sugar in the urine, with the use of hydrochloric acid as one of the reagents.

1870   ERNEST MARCEL LABBÉ born.
A French physiologist from Paris who was the first to give a full description of chromaffin cell tumors of the adrenal medulla.

1870 GEORGE LUDWIG ZUELZER born.
A German chemist who gave the first subcutaneous injection of pancreatic extract to a 50-year-old diabetic patient (1906), producing a temporary recovery, and patented his preparation in 1912.

1871 ERWIN PAYR born.
A professor of surgery at Leipzig in Germany who described a fold of the peritoneum over the splenic flexure of the colon (Payr membrane).

1871 HOWARD DAVIS HASKIN born.
An American surgeon who devised a test for urinary proteins using acetic acid and sodium chloride as reagents.

1871 SIR ROBERT HUTCHINSON born.
A physician at the Hospital for Sick Children at Great Ormond Street who was the first to isolate globulin and described suprarenal sarcoma of children which led to secondary growths in the skull.

1872 HUGH CABOT born.
An American urologist and specialist in the treatment of hypospadias who devised an operation for undescended testis.

1872 Arteriosclerotic atrophy of the kidney was described by WILLIAM WITHEY GULL and HENRY GAWEN SUTTON of London.

1873 EUGENE LINDSAY OPIE born.
A Virginia pathologist who suggested the presence of an antidiabetic substance in the islets of Langerhans of the pancreas (1903), while professor at the John Hopkins Hospital at Baltimore.

1873   RUPERT WATERHOUSE born.
An English physician at the Royal National Hospital for
Rheumatic Diseases who described suprarenal apoplexy as the
cause of Waterhouse–Friderichsen syndrome.

1873   FRANCIS RANDALL HAGNER born.
An American urologist who designed an inflatable rubber bag
placed in the urethra to arrest bleeding during prostatectomy,
and an operation for acute epididymitis (Hagner operation).

1873   EUGENE HAHN, a German surgeon, devised an operation for
movable kidney, and a modified cannula with a sponge for use
in endotracheal anesthesia.

1874   The Bottini operation, where a channel was made
through the prostate with galvanocautery for the treatment
of enlarged prostate (prostatectomy), was designed by
Italian surgeon, ENRICO BOTTINI.

1874   DANIEL JOSEPH MCCARTHY born.
A New York urologist who designed a panendoscope, prostatic
electrotome, and several other instruments.

1874   ALFRED BAKER SPALDING born.
An American gynecologist from San Francisco who described
an operation for uterine prolapse.

1874   The secretion theory for renal function was put forward by
German professor of physiology, RUDOLF PETER HEINRICH
HEIDENHAIN.

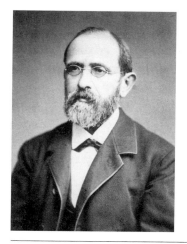

Rudolf Peter Heinrich Heidenhain
(1834–1897)

1874   Contraction of the abdominal muscles on compression of the
testicles (testicular reflex) was described by Swiss surgeon,
EMILE THEODOR KOCHER.

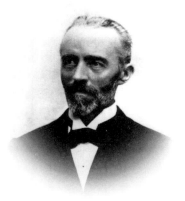

Emile Theodor Kocher
(1841–1917)

1874   Acetonemia as a cause of diabetic coma was recognized by
German professor of surgery, ADOLF KUSSMAUL.

1874 WILLIAM GEORGE MACCALLUM born.
A Canadian-born pathologist who suggested the
association between lesions of the islets of Langerhans
and glycosuria.

1875 Otto Rossel born.
A physician from Switzerland who detected occult blood in feces
using Barbados aloin and other reagents (Rossel test).

1875 A urinary bladder tumor was first excised through the
abdominal route by Austrian surgeon, CHRISTIAN ALBERT
THEODOR BILLROTH.

1875 WILHELM FALTA born.
An Austrian physician who studied endocrine and metabolic
disorders, including diabetes mellitus, and wrote *The Diseases
of the Bloodglands*.

1876 JOHN TIMOTHY GERAGHTY born.
An American surgeon who described a new method of
perineal prostatectomy.

1876 MAURICE FAVRE born.
A French dermatologist who made important
contributions to the understanding of syphilis, especially
lymphogranuloma inguinale, which he separated from
other venereal diseases.

1876 The intestinal parasitic roundworm that causes diarrhea
(*Strongyloides stercoralis*) was first described by
LOUIS NORMAND in Cochin, China.

1876   JOHN JAMES RICKARD MACLEOD born.
A Scottish professor of physiology who carried out important research on diabetes, published *Physiology and Biochemistry in Modern Medicine*, and shared the Nobel Prize for the discovery of insulin.

1876   JOHN SWIFT JOLY born.
A London urologist who devised an irrigating urethroscope, also used for cystoscopy, pioneered the use of radium for cancer treatment, and devised the Dublin method of radiotherapy.

1877   A description of familial nephrogenic diabetes insipidus was given by London physician, SAMUEL JONES GEE in *Contributions to the History of Polydipsia*.

1877   The first nephrectomy for malignant disease of the kidney was carried out by CARL JOHANN AUGUST LANGENBUCH of Berlin, Germany.

1877   The first electrically-lit cystoscope was devised by Berlin urologist, MAX NITZE.

1878   The fungus *Actinomyces israelii* was discovered by German urologist, JAMES ADOLPH ISRAEL.

1878   ERNEST LOWENSTEIN born.
A Viennese pathologist who (with Danish bacteriologist, ORLA JENSEN), prepared the Lowenstein–Jensen medium, used to culture *Mycobacterium tuberculosis*.

1878   HENRY ORLANDO MARCY, American surgeon from Massachusetts, introduced antiseptic sutures in the surgical treatment of hernia.

1878 A case of primary cancer of the ureter established by microscopic diagnosis was reported by a Swedish physician, P JOHANN WISING.

1878 HANS ZINSSER born.
An American bacteriologist who worked on allergy, virus size, typhus and causes of rheumatic fever, differentiated epidemic from endemic ricketsial typhus, and wrote *Rats, Lice and History.*

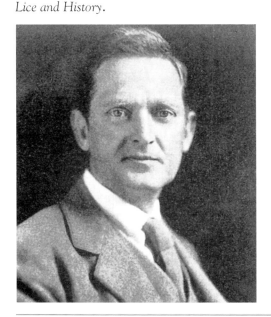

Hans Zinsser
(1878–1940)

1878 FRANK SEYMOUR KIDD born.
A London urologist who designed an operating cystoscope (Kidd cystoscope) with an electrode, for diathermy of bladder tumors.

1879 Winckel disease, characterized by icterus, bloody urine and hemorrhage with a fatal outcome in neonates, was described by German gynecologist, FRANZ KARL LUDWIG VON WINCKEL.

1879   HANS CHRISTIAN JACOBAEUS born.
A Stockholm surgeon who used a modified cystoscope to perform cautery division of pleural adhesions, which led directly to the development of the thoracoscope and other similar instruments.

1880   ALBERT A EPSTEIN born.
An American physician who made important contributions to renal disease and diabetes, including a microchemical method for estimating sugar in the blood, and described Epstein syndrome.

1880   The paraurethral glands of the female (Skene glands) were described by ALEXANDER J C SKENE, an American gynecologist of Scottish origin.

1880   A procedure for nephrolithotomy, where the renal stone was removed through a lumbar incision, was performed by SIR HENRY MORRIS of London.

1880   ERNST LAQUEUR born.
A Dutch physician and urologist who was one of the discoverers of testosterone, and also of estrogenic activity in male urine.

1880   ARTHUR C ALPORT born.
He is remembered for an eponymous syndrome of hereditary nephritis which is often accompanied by sensorineural hearing loss, lenticonus, and maculopathy.

1881   HANS REITER born.
A German physician from Leipzig who described urethritis, conjunctivitis and arthritis (Reiter disease) while working as an army surgeon during the First World War.

1881 'Nephrosis' was used by FRIEDRICH VON MÜLLER to refer to primary degenerative forms of Bright disease, and to differentiate it from diseases of an inflammatory nature.

1881 The Fehling operation, used in the treatment of prolapse of the uterus, was devised by German gynecologist, HERMANN JOHANNES KARL FEHLING.

1881 Nephropexy, an operation to fix a movable kidney, was performed by German surgeon, EUGENE HAHN.

1881 WILLIAM ROBERTS of Manchester observed the rod-shaped bacteria in the urine, symptomatic of bacteriuria.

1881 A study of the mechanics and pattern of urine flow was achieved by the Italian physiologists ANGELO MOSSO and PELLCANI, who devised a manometer to record the intravesical pressure at rest and during micturition.

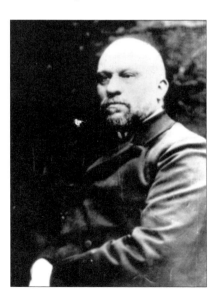

Angelo Mosso
(1846–1910)

1882   WILLIAM EDWARD GALLIE born.
A Canadian professor of surgery who introduced fascial sutures for surgery of inguinal hernia.

1883   HENRY JACOB BIGELOW of Harvard modified CIVIALE'S lithotrite to crush larger and heavier stones. He removed the fragments with a special metal catheter, to the outer end of which was attached a rubber bulb evacuator with a glass container below to receive the fragments.

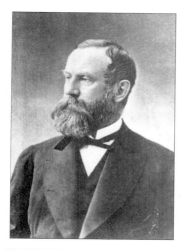

Henry Jacob Bigelow
(1818–1890)

1883   Beta-oxybutyric acid in urine was discovered by a German physical chemist, ERNEST STADELMAN.

1883   Retrorenal fascia (Zuckerkandl fascia) was described by Hungarian-born anatomist, EMIL ZUCKERKANDL. He also wrote an important monograph on the pathology and anatomy of the accessory sinuses.

1883   Renal osteodystrophy in patients with chronic renal disease (renal rickets) was first described by RICHARD CLEMENT LUCAS of Guy's Hospital in London.

1883   HUGH MACLEAN born.
A professor of medicine at the University of London and
St Thomas' Hospital who designed the urea concentration
test for renal function.

1883   The Ehrlich test for bile pigments in urine was devised by
German bacteriologist and Nobel laureate, PAUL EHRLICH.

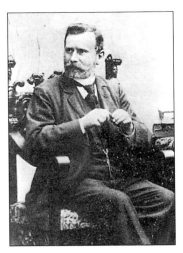

Paul Ehrlich
(1854–1915)

1883   The Gram stain for bacteria was discovered by
HANS CHRISTIAN JOACHIM GRAM of Denmark, while
working on methods for double-staining kidney sections.

1884   The origin and nature of hypernephroma or renal cell
carcinoma (Grawitz tumor) was first studied by German
pathologist, PAUL ALBERT GRAWITZ.

1884   BURRILL B CROHN born.
An American physician who presented a paper on a new,
regional disease consisting of abdominal pain, diarrhea,
and a mass often in the lower quadrant (Crohn disease, or
regional ileitis).

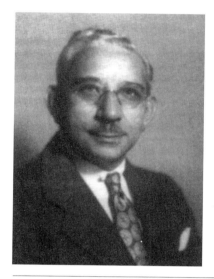

Burrill B Crohn (1884–1983)

1885   Scottish physician, SIR THOMAS RICHARD FRASER, investigated kombe poison from Africa, and demonstrated its therapeutic effect in dropsy.

1885   The downward displacement of the viscera (enteropathy) in association with neurasthenia (Glenard syndrome) was described by French physician, FRANTZ GLENARD.

1885   ADOLF EDELMAN born.
        An Austrian physician who was the first to describe anemia in chronic infections, in addition to devising a test for urobilin in urine.

1885   A chronic relapsing condition of the colon (ulcerative colitis) was described as 'acute extensive ulcerations of the colon' by SIR WILLIAM ALLCHIN of London.

1885   The occurrence of acid intoxication in renal failure (renal acidosis) was observed by RUDOLF VON JAKSCH, a Czech physician from Prague.

1886 Operative treatment for hydronephrosis was performed by
FRIEDRICH TRENDELENBURG of Germany.

1886 HENRY ARNOLD KIRKPATRICK born.
A Dublin surgeon who described an operation for femoral
hernia through a midline extraperitoneal approach, and
devised the posterior approach for excision of thoracic
sympathetic ganglia and the sympathetic trunk.

1886 A method of estimating creatinine in blood was devised by
MAX JAFFE, a biochemist from Königsberg, Germany.

1886 CHARLES FREDERICK MORRIS SAINT born.
He described the Saint triad, consisting of gallbladder disease,
diverticulosis and hiatus hernia, and was a South African
physician at Groote Schuur Hospital.

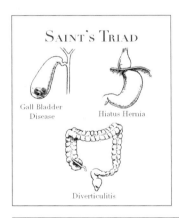

Illustration of the Saint triad

1886 CHESTER JEFFERSON FARMER born.
A Chicago chemist who developed microchemical assay
methods for urea, creatinine, and other substances.

1886 'Ballotement', a valuable sign for tumors of the kidney, was described by French scientist, JEAN C F GUYON.

1886 An enlarged deformed kidney (Formad kidney) was observed in some cases of chronic alcoholism by American physician, HENRY F FORMAD.

1887 ALFRED E FRANK born.
A German physician who identified diabetes insipidus as being due to a lesion of the posterior pituitary, and described non-thrombocytopenic purpura (Frank capillary toxicosis).

1887 Nitze's cystoscope was fitted with Edison's electric light by both HARTWIG of Berlin and LEITER of Vienna.

1887 Irish surgeon, CHARLES BENT BALL, described a radical cure for abdominal hernia, the Ball operation, described the rectal valves (Ball valves) in *The Rectum and Anus, their Diseases and Treatment*, and devised an operation for the relief of pruritis.

1887 SIR WILLIAM HENEAGE OGILVIE born.
He was a London surgeon at Guy's Hospital, and described functional obstruction of the large bowel in elderly patients (Ogilvie syndrome).

1887 The area in the anterior wall of the vagina in contact with the base of the bladder and free of vaginal rugae was described by KAREL PAWLIK, a gynecologist from Prague.

1888 Cancer of the pancreas was described by Swiss physician LOUIS BARD.

1888 An important treatise on surgical diseases of the bladder and prostate was published by JEAN C FELIX GUYON of Paris, the founder of modern genitourinary surgery, who published his lectures on urology a few years earlier.

1888 An operative treatment for rectal prolapse was described by Polish surgeon, JOHANN VON MIKULICZ-RADECKI.

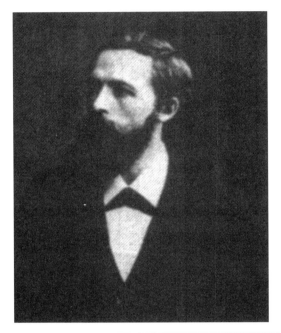

Johann von
Mikulicz-Radecki
(1850–1905)

1888 Polymyalgia rheumatica was described as senile rheumatic gout by W BRUCE in the *British Medical Journal*.

1888 The fibromuscular mass found between the coccyx and the anus in the perineum (Symington anococcygial body) was described by Scottish anatomist, JOHNSON SYMINGTON.

1888 Congenital megacolon (Hirschsprung disease) was first described by Danish pediatrician, HARALD HIRSCHSPRUNG.

1889 ELI KINNERLEY MARSHALL born.
A pharmacologist at the Johns Hopkins Hospital who demonstrated the secretory function of the renal convoluted tubule, using phenolsulfonephthalein.

1889 The first systematic experiments to show that pancreatectomy led to diabetes mellitus were carried out by Nobel laureates, JOSEF VON MERING and OSKAR MINKOWSKI.

1889 A rash (erythema gluteale or Jacquet disease), due to irritation by ammonia in the urine in the area where the napkin or diaper is applied, was described by Paris pediatrician, LEONARD MARIE LUCIEN JACQUET.

1890 The Manchester operation for uterine prolapse, involving high amputation of the cervix and repair of the anterior and posterior vaginal walls, was devised by ARCHIBALD DONALD of Manchester.

1890 An acute rapidly progressive form of diabetes mellitus (Hirschfeld disease) was first described by German physician, FELIX HIRSCHFELD.

1890 Tenderness was localized in the right side over the inflamed gallbladder in cholecystitis (Courvoisier sign), by LUDWIG GEORG COURVOISIER, a surgeon from Switzerland.

1890   Urology became a separate study course from
general surgery, and the first professor of urology was
JEAN C FELIX GUYON in Paris.

1891   GEORGE LIGNAC born.
A Dutch pathologist who studied cystine metabolic anomalies
and their effects on the kidneys, and the effects of benzol as a
leukemogenic agent.

1891   American urologist, FREDERIC EUGENE BASIL FOLEY born.
He designed a pneumatic cold punch resectoscope for
removal of the prostate through the urethra, a plastic
operation for hydronephrosis, and a double-lumened
retention catheter with a balloon on the end to keep it in
the bladder (1933).

1891   The abnormal position of the suprarenal glands in
certain patients was described by German pathologist,
FELIX JACOB MARCHAND.

1892   Solute concentrations of urine and blood were first
compared to assess renal function by HEINRICH DRESSLER of
Germany.

1892   An important study on the gallstone was made by Swiss
professor of clinical medicine, BERNARD NAUNYN, who
published his findings in *Klinik der Cholelithiasis*, and
later advocated drainage of the bile duct in cases of
cholecystotomy.

1892   The two-stage operation for carcinoma of the colon was devised by German surgeon, OSCAR THORVALD BLOCH.

1892   Bladder cancer was first linked to a chemical compound involved in fuchsin manufacture by German surgeon, LUDWIG REHN.

1893   The cell mass found in the male urethra was described by ALBERT VON BRUNN.

1893   An operative procedure for uncomplicated femoral hernia and an another for radical cure of inguinal hernia were described by EDOARDO BASSINI of Italy.

1893   The cutaneous areas of the sensory nerve roots related to visceral organs were mapped by SIR HENRY HEAD, a London neurologist.

1893   Glycosuria during increased epinephrine secretion was noted by F BLUM.

1893   The catheterization of male ureters was first done by JAMES BROWN of Johns Hopkins Hospital.

1894   HAMILTON BAILEY born.
A London surgeon who designed a suprapubic trocar for puncturing the urinary bladder.

1894   Chicago surgeon, FREDERIC FENGER, devised the Fenger operation for relief of ureteral stricture causing hydronephrosis.

1894   British physiologists, HUGH KERR ANDERSON and JOHN
NEWPORT LANGLEY, used the term 'axon reflex' to denote
the reflex response of the urinary bladder to nerve
stimulation.

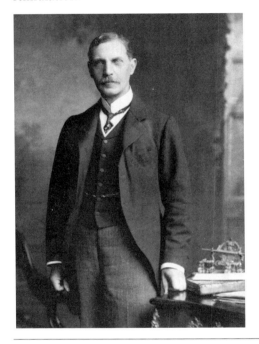

John Newport
Langley (1852–1925)

1894   The White operation, castration for hypertrophy of the
prostate, was devised by Philadelphia surgeon,
J WILLIAM WHITE.

1894   EUGENE FULLER of New York was credited with being the first
to describe a technique for the removal of a prostatic adenoma
via the suprapubic route.

1894   Peritoneal dialysis was investigated by Dutch physiologist,
HARTOG JAKOB HAMBURGER.

1895   Early diagnosis of stone disease became possible after the discovery of X-rays, and in 1896 MCINTYRE of Glasgow visualized a kidney stone with this method.

1895   The Masset test for detection of bile pigments in urine, by adding sulfuric acid and potassium nitrate to give a distinctive green color, was devised by French physician, ALFRED AUGUST MASSET.

1895   Cryoscopic examination of urine was first introduced by Hungarian physician, ALEXANDER VON SANDOR KORANYI.

1895   GEORGE OLIVER and EDWARD SHARPEY-SCHÄFER from England demonstrated that extracts of the suprarenal gland, when injected intravenously, produced a contraction of the arteries and acceleration of the heart rate, thereby increasing blood pressure.

1895   The treatment of inguinal hernia with overlapping sutures (Andrews operation) was designed by American surgeon, EDWARD WYLLYS ANDREWS.

1896   Renal decapsulation was performed by American comparative anatomist, R Harrison, and revived by New York surgeon, GEORGE MICHAEL EDEBOHLS, seven years later.

1896   Ureterosigmoidostomy for urinary diversion was performed by French surgeon, HENRI CHAPUT.

1896   PHILIP SHOWALTER HENCH born.
        An American physician who noticed that surgery, pregnancy and starvation stimulated the adrenal cortex and improved rheumatoid arthritis, and later noted the effect of cortisone in treatment, for which he received the Nobel Prize.

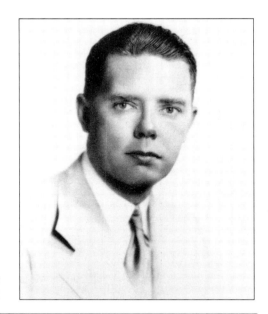

Philip Showalter
Hench (1896–1965)

1897 MANES KARTAGENER born.
A physician from Switzerland who described a hereditary
disorder involving bronchiectasis with transposition of the
viscera (Kartagener syndrome).

1898 JOHN JACOB ABEL of Johns Hopkins Medical School
constructed the first membrane for artificial kidneys, was
the first to obtain a crystalline form of insulin (1926), and
also first to extract epinephrine, hirudin, specific amino acids,
and posterior pituitary hormones from the blood, and
used the leech to prevent the clotting of blood during his
experiments on artificial kidneys (1910).

1898 The X-linked condition, Fabry disease, resulting in renal
failure, corneal opacities and multiple skin lesions, was
described by German dermatologist, J FABRY.

1898   ARTHUR MAURICE FISHBERG born.
A New York physician who devised a concentration test for
renal function.

1898   A monograph on diabetes, *Der Diabetes Mellitus*, was
published by BERNARD NAUNYN, professor of clinical
medicine in Strasbourg.

1898   A method of obtaining urine samples from each kidney
separately was described by Chicago surgeon, MALCOLM LA
SALLE HARRIS.

1899   A book on embryonic tumor of the kidney (nephroblastoma,
or Wilms tumor) was published by German professor of
surgery, MAX WILMS.

1899   FELIX TURYN born.
A Polish physician from Warsaw who described pain in
the gluteal region if the great toe is bent in cases of
sciatica.

1900   The first description of Ebstein anomaly in America was given
by WILLIAM GEORGE MACCALLUM, a pathologist at the Johns
Hopkins Hospital in Baltimore.

1900   SIR HANS ADOLF KREBS born.
A German-born British biochemist and Nobel laureate
(1953) who described metabolism in the urea and citric
acid cycles.

1900   Dilatation of the ureteral orifice as treatment for ureteric
calculi was first performed by Baltimore urologist,
HOWARD ATWOOD KELLY.

1900 SIR ARCHIBALD HECTOR MCINDOE born.
A New Zealand-born London surgeon who described a
procedure for reconstruction of the urethra with a dermal
graft, and devised an operation for construction of the vagina
in cases of its congenital absence.

1901 JOKICHI TAKAMINE of Japan obtained the first pure chemical
form of epinephrine while working in New Jersey.

1901 CHARLES BRENTON HUGGINS born.
A Canadian-born US surgeon and Nobel laureate (1966)
who pioneered hormone treatment of cancer, and
investigated the physiology of the male urinogenital tract.

1902 JOHANNES ZOON, a Dutch dermatologist, born.
Zoon balanitis is a benign condition of the foreskin
which causes irritation and some fixation. It is
characterized by small erythematous papular lesions
which appear as reddish brown discoloration, and is cured
by circumcision.

1902 Radical testicular surgery involving the removal of the lumbar
lymph nodes and spermatic vein was described by
Philadelphia surgeon, JOHN BINGHAM ROBERTS.

1902 EMIL FISCHER received the Nobel Prize for work on proteins
and amino acids. In 1903 he synthesized Veronal, and other
soporific urea derivatives. He investigated and named
'purine', and identified uric acid as a trioxypurine, important
in understanding the metabolism of gout.

1902   ARNE W K TISELIUS born.
A Swedish chemist from Stockholm and Nobel laureate
(1948) who isolated several viruses and separated and
identified amino acids, sugars and other molecules,
using activated charcoal, silica, cellulose, and ion
exchange chromatography.

1902   The first kidney transplant was performed when a dog's
kidney was transplanted into a goat's neck by EMERICH
ULLMAN, an Austrian surgeon.

1903   A method of estimating specific gravity of small amounts of
urine was described by New York physician, GEORGE
ALEXANDER DE SANTOS.

1903   Widespread deposition of cystine crystals was described in
children who died of resistant rickets, polyuria, renal
glycosuria, and acidosis (Fanconi syndrome), by Swiss
physiologist, EMIL ABERHALDEN.

1904   HUGH HAMPSON YOUNG, a prominent American
urologist, devised a technique of prostatectomy using a
perineal approach, developed the radical prostatectomy
in 1906, invented cystoscopes, and operated for
retrourethral fistula.

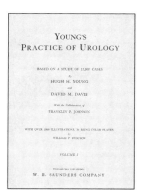

Frontispiece of Young's
Practice of Urology

1904   SIR GEORGE WHITE PICKERING born.
        A professor of medicine at Oxford who studied hypertension,
        and noted the protein nature of renin and its role in
        hypertension.

1904   The term 'hypernephroma' was introduced by German
        pathologist, OTTO LUBARSCH.

1905   British physiologists, WILLIAM MADDOCKS BAYLISS and
        ERNEST HENRY STARLING obtained a substance from the
        intestinal mucous membrane which had a remote action
        on the pancreas, which they named 'secretin'.

1905   HANS HELLER born.
        An Austrian endocrinologist who studied water metabolism
        and neurohypophysial hormones.

1905   The relationship between sex organs and suprarenal
        glands was described by WILLIAM BULLOCK and
        JAMES HARRY SEQUIRA.

1905   The Rabe test to detect albumin in urine using
        trichloroacetic acid was devised by German physician,
        GUSTAV RAABE.

1905   The term 'azotemia' was used
        by French microbiologist, GEORGES
        F I WIDAL, to denote a syndrome
        that resulted from retention of
        nitrogenous materials, normally
        eliminated by the kidneys.

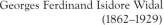

Georges Ferdinand Isidore Widal
(1862–1929)

1906   LUIS FREDERICO LELOIR born.
        A French-born Argentinian biochemist who worked on
        diabetes and the adrenals, noted the proteolytic action of
        renin from kidneys leading to production of angiotensin, and
        discovered glucose-1-phosphate kinase.

1906   The radiological method of visualization of the renal
        tract (pyelography) was introduced by ALEXANDER VON
        LICHTENBERG of Germany.

1906   HIRSCH WOLF SULKOWITCH born.
        A Boston physician who devised the Sulkowitch test for
        detecting calcium in urine.

1906   ALFRED L GRAY, an American physician, introduced
        radiotherapy as an alternative procedure in the
        treatment of bladder cancer and subsequently in
        prostatic cancer therapy.

1907   Hematuria with focal glomerular lesions in the kidney due to
        minute bacterial emboli from endocardial vegetations in
        bacterial endocarditis (embolic nephritis) was observed by
        MAX H F LOEHLEIN of Leipzig.

1907   HANS SELYE born.
        A Canadian physician who carried out important work on
        hormonal interactions involving the adrenal and pituitary
        glands and the hypothalamus, in osteoblast multiplication,
        bone formation, and blood sugar level.

1908   The Rothera test which detects acetone in the urine was devised by an Australian biochemist, ARTHUR CECIL HAMEL ROTHERA.

1908   Abdominoperineal resection of the rectum for rectal carcinoma (Miles operation) was devised by English surgeon, WILLIAM ERNEST MILES.

1909   Some of the first detailed studies on the urinary passages were written by Cuban-born French physician, JOAQUÍN DOMINGUEZ ALBARRÁN. He described treatment for hydronephrosis in 1895.

1909   The Hartmann operation for the removal of upper rectum or sigmoid in cancer, together with closure of the rectal stump and establishment of colostomy, was described by French surgeon, HENRI HARTMANN.

1909   Irrigation and observation of the bladder was made possible by the Brown–Buerger cystoscope, devised by LEO BUERGER, a US urologist from Vienna, in collaboration with F TILDER BROWN.

1909   ELDON J GARDNER born.
An American geneticist who described the hereditary autosomal dominant condition associated with colonic polyposis and increased risk of carcinoma (Gardner syndrome).

1910   The phenolsulfonphthalein test, to estimate renal functions, was devised by LEONARD GEORGE ROWNTREE, director of the Philadelphia Medical Institute, and another American, JOHN TIMOTHY GERAGHTY.

1910 The formula to determine the concentrating power of the kidney, using urea and blood ratios and known as the Ambard coefficient, was proposed by French physiologist, Leo Ambard, in Strasbourg.

1910 John Jacob Abel of Johns Hopkins University used leeches to prevent the clotting of blood during his experiments on artificial kidneys.

1911 Willem Johan Kolff born.
A Dutch-born American physician and pioneer of the artificial kidney who constructed the first rotating drum artificial kidney, in wartime Holland, and developed the artificial kidney and a heart–lung machine after moving to America.

1911 The Coffey operation, in which ureters are transplanted into the colon, was designed by surgeon from Portland, Oregon, Robert Calvin Coffey.

1911 Norepinephrine was discovered by George Barger and Henry Dale at Edinburgh University and the National Institute for Medical Research.

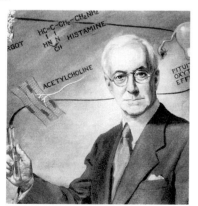

Sir Henry Hallett Dale
(1875–1968)

1911 Premature separation of a normally implanted placenta, accompanied by albuminuria, azotemia and shock (Couvelaire syndrome) was described by French obstetrician, ALEXANDRE COUVELAIRE.

1912 Azotemia, produced by an extrarenal cause such as cholera (prerenal uremia), was first observed by GEORGE FROIN and PIERRE MARIE of Paris.

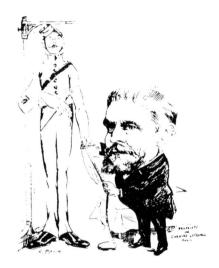

Cartoon of Pierre Marie (1853–1940)

1912 German organic chemist and Nobel laureate, HEINRICH OTTO WIELAnd, demonstrated that bile acids were steroids, based on the structure of cholesterol.

1913 Starvation as a method of lowering blood sugars in treatment for diabetes (Allen starvation) was proposed by FREDERICK MADISON ALLEN, a Boston diabetologist.

1913 New York urologist, MAX HUHNER, estimated the motility and the number of spermatozoa during postcoital examination.

1913 The peritoneal band extending from the mesocolon to the duodenojejunal flexure (Pringle band) was described by Dublin surgeon, SETON SYDNEY PRINGLE.

1913 The term 'lipid nephrosis' was first used by German physician, FRITZ MUNK.

1914 FREDERICK C BARTTER born.
An American physician best known for his description of Bartter syndrome, diminished sodium resorption of the kidney leading to hypokalemic alkalosis.

1914 Experimental studies on renal grafts (renal transplantation) were carried out by Nobel laureate, ALEXIS CARREL, an American surgeon and pioneer in the field of transplantation.

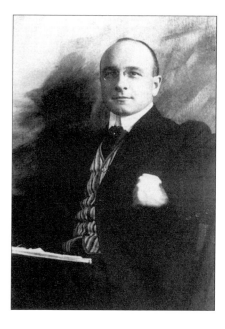

Alexis Carrel
(1883–1944)

1914   Barium enema as a diagnostic test in radiology was introduced, thereby making the recognition of colonic diverticular disease more common.

1914   The nitric test, to detect urinary tract infection, was devised by J CRUICKSHANK and J MOYES of England.

1915   The rise of phosphate levels in the blood of patients with renal failure (hyperphosphatemia) was first observed by GREENWALD.

1916   Reiter disease, characterized by urethritis, conjunctivitis, and arthritis, was described by German bacteriologist, HANS REITER of the German Medical Corps.

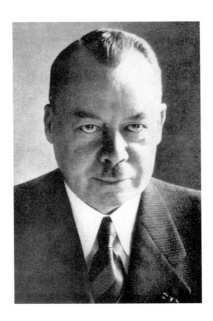

Hans Reiter (1881–1969)

1916   THOMAS ADDIS, a US physician from Scotland, published studies on the kidney and urine excretion with G Barnett of Stamford University. He also studied the effect of dietary protein on renal function and its importance in management of renal disease.

The Addis count, a quantitative enumeration of urinary cellular excretion in a 12-hour urine specimen, is used to follow the progress of known renal disease.

1916   The rise of uric acid in the blood which precedes the rise of urea in renal failure was noted by VICTOR CARLYL MYERS.

1917   The Mayo Clinic was established and the Mayo Foundation for Medical Education and Research was endowed. The names of the three Mayo brothers are also associated with the Mayo operation for umbilical hernia, Mayo kidney incision, and Mayo scissors.

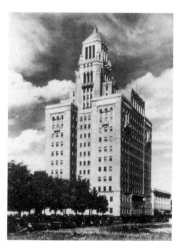

The Mayo Clinic
in Rochester

1917 Kidney functions based on both secretory and mechanical theories were explained by ARTHUR ROBERTSON CUSHNY, a British pharmacologist.

1917 Fouchet reagent, used in testing for the presence of bilirubin in urine, was prepared by French chemist and physician, ANDRE FOUCHET.

1918 An operative method for femoral hernia (Dowden operation) was devised by Edinburgh surgeon, JOHN WHEELER DOWDEN.

1918 Japanese professor KENJI TAKANAGI from Tokyo University devised a modified cystoscope.

1919 An early method of surgical treatment for uterine prolapse was devised by American obstetrician and gynecologist, ALFRED BAKER SPALDING.

1919 Associated with acute nephritis and hemoptysis, Goodpasture syndrome was described in an 18-year-old male by American virologist, ERNEST WILLIAM GOODPASTURE.

1919 Experimental rejuvenation by means of a testicular transplant was reported by a French physiologist of Russian origin, SERGE VORONOFF.

1919 JOSEPH EDWARD MURRAY born.
An American surgeon, Nobel laureate (1990) and pioneer in renal transplantation who performed the first renal transplant between identical twins (1954) and, later, non-identical twins (1961).

1920   BARUJ BENACERRAF born.
A Venezuelan-born American immunologist and Nobel laureate (1980) who studied immunological responses to diseased cells, and organ transplantation.

1920   A measure of functions of the kidneys (urea concentration) was devised by HUGH MACLEAN and OWEN LAMBART DE WESSELOW.

1920   The hippuric acid synthesis test (where benzoic acid combines with glycol in the kidney to form hippuric acid) was used to test for renal functions by ÉMILE ACHARD and CHAPELLE of Paris. Achard coined the term 'paratyphoid fever', and wrote on encephalitis lethargica, and edema in Bright disease.

1921   Radiological visualization of the kidneys by injecting air into the retroperitoneal space (retroperitoneal pneumatography) was devised by ROSSENTEIN and CARELLI.

1922   Erythrocytosis, caused by renal disease was described by German physician, FELIX GAISBOCK.

1923   The highly vasculated area on the colon, between the colic and superior rectal arteries (Sudeck critical point), was described by PAUL SUDECK, a surgeon in Hamburg.

1923   Glucagon, a hormone in extract of pancreas which causes a rise in blood sugar, was discovered by JOHN R MURLIN and C P KIMBALL at the University of Rochester.

1923 FREDERICK GRANT BANTING and JOHN MCLEOD won the Nobel Prize for Physiology or Medicine for the discovery of insulin.

1923 The fungus causing thrush, *Candida albicans*, was named by CHRISTINE BERKHOUT from the University of Delft, Holland.

1924 The presence of amino acids in urine and cystine crystals in the bone marrow of patients with cystinosis was demonstrated by Dutch pathologist, G O E LIGNAC.

1925 Surgical hernia following the surgical incision of the abdomen was studied by American surgeon, ARTHUR MARRIOT SHIPLEY, who described a method of closure.

1925 DANIEL ALAGILLE born.
A French pediatrician who described multiple abnormalities associating neonatal cholestasis prolonged during childhood and adulthood due to paucity of interlobular bile ducts (Alagille syndrome).

1925 The causative organism of gonorrhea *(Neisseria gonorrhoeae)* was discovered by ALBERT NEISSER, while he was a research assistant at the Berlin Hospital.

1926 SELMAR ASCHHEIM and BERNHARDT ZONDEK of Berlin found a substance in urine of pregnant women similar to gonadotropic hormone from the anterior pituitary, later named anterior pituitary-like hormone.

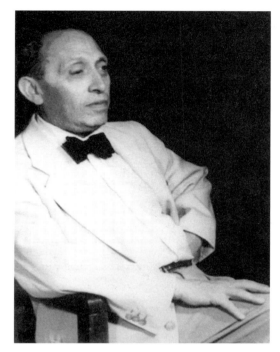

Bernhardt Zondek
(1891–1966)

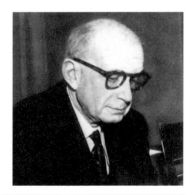

Selmar Aschheim
(1878–1965)

1926   Adrenal insufficiency and hypothyroidism (Schmidt
        syndrome) was described by MARTIN BENNO SCHMIDT
        of Germany.

1927 KENNETH F FAIRLEY born.
An Australian physician from Melbourne who described a bladder washout test to determine the site of urinary infection (Fairley test).

1928 Hypervitaminosis D, associated with metastatic calcification and renal calculi following high intake of ergosterol in experimental animals, was first demonstrated independently by PFANNENSTEIN, and KREITMER.

1928 Irritable bowel syndrome, or spastic colon, was described by JOHN ALFRED RYLE, a physician at Guy's Hospital.

1928 The urea clearance test for renal function was devised by Paris physician, LEO AMBARD, American physician, FRANKLIN C MCLEAN and San Francisco physician, THOMAS ADDIS.

1929 The association between polyuria of diabetes insipidus and the action of the posterior pituitary extract was noted by British pharmacologist, ERNEST BASIL VERNEY.

1929 The first steroid hormone, estrone, was extracted in a pure state from the urine obtained during pregnancy, independently by EDWARD DOISY and ADOLF F J BUTENANDT.

1929 The ability of the vertebrate kidney to secrete foreign substances was demonstrated by ELI KENNERLEY MARSHALL, an American pharmacologist from the Johns Hopkins Hospital in Baltimore.

1929   Intravenous urography was introduced by German-born American urologist, MOSES SWICK.

1930   H B ANDERSON reported the first case of hypoglycemia in a patient with an adrenal tumor.

1930   The classification of nephritis, based on the hemorrhagic nature and nephrosclerosis, was proposed by American biochemist, DONALD D VAN SLYKE and colleagues.

1930   The first active cortical extract from the renal glands (corticosteroid) was prepared by WILBER WILLIS SWINGLE and JOSEPH JOHN PFIFFNER.

1930   B SHAPIRO of Germany started treating undescended testis (cryptorchidism) with an anterior pituitary-like substance isolated from the urine of pregnant women.

1930   ARTHUR M FISHBERG of Mount Sinai Hospital, New York classified nephritis into various forms, including focal glomerular nephritis and acute interstitial nephritis.

1930   A test using copper sulfate solution in the detection of sugar in the blood and urine (Benedict solution) was devised by STANLEY ROSSITER BENEDICT.

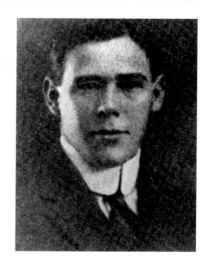

Stanley Rossiter Benedict
(1884–1936)

1932 A classification for rectal carcinoma was proposed by London pathologist, CUTHBERT DUKES (Dukes classification).

1932 A measure of renal function (xylose excretion test) was devised by ELLA S FISHBERG and FRIEDLAND.

1932 Dutch physicians, ERNST LACQUER, E DINGEMANSE and S E JONGH, observed estrogenic activity in male urine.

1933 A technique for recording internal body images at a predetermined plane using X-rays (tomography) was described by German physician, D L BARTELINK.

1933 Hyperinsulinism was described by SEELE HARRIS of America.

1933 Hippuran, an agent in urography, was introduced by MOSES SWICK.

1933 DEREK DENNY-BROWN and ROBERTSON designed a catheter, manometer and a moving strip of bromide paper to measure and record bladder and sphincter behavior.

1934 A quantitative method of estimating urinary sediments was devised by San Francisco physician, HENRY GIBBONS.

1934 American biochemist, JOSEPH HYRAM ROE, devised a colorimetric test for fructose in urine and blood (fructosuria).

1934   The production of renal hypertension by clamping the renal artery was shown by HARRY GOLDBLATT, an American experimental pathologist, with J LYNCH and R F HANZAL.

1935   Mandelic acid was first used in the treatment of urinary tract infections by MAX LEONHARD ROSENHEIM.

1935   G F CAWHILL used radiological visualization of adrenal tumors by introducing air around the perinephric area.

1935   M BURGER and W BRANDT discovered the humoral hyperglycemic action of glucagon.

1936   Cortisone was isolated independently by Nobel laureates, TADEUS REICHSTEIN, EDWARD CALVIN KENDALL and OSKAR PAUL WINTERSTEINER.

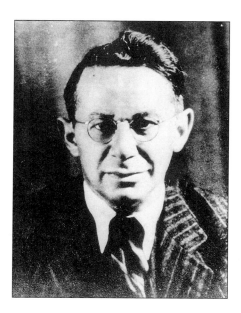

Tadeus Reichstein
(1897–1996)

1936 Peculiar spherical masses in the central portion of glomerular globules (Kimmelsteil–Wilson lesion) were first described (intercapillary glomerular sclerosis) in eight patients with diabetes by German–American pathologist, PAUL KIMMELSTEIL.

1936 The lymphatic spread of carcinoma of the prostate to the bones (Warren theory) was proposed by American physician, SHIELDS WARREN.

1937 Orogenital ulceration (Behçet syndrome) was described by Turkish dermatologist, HALUSHI BEHÇET, who wrote *Syphilis and Related Skin Diseases.*

1937 A contrast medium was first injected directly into the renal arteries by a Spanish physician, REYNALDO DOS SANTOS.

1937 The urographic appearance of the kidneys in renal papillary necrosis was described by G W GUNTHER of Stuttgart, Germany.

1938 Rare renal hemangioma tumors were found by ELEXIUS THOMPSON BELL, a pathologist at the University of Minnesota.

1938 Metastatic lesions of prostate cancer were shown to cause elevation of serum levels of acid phosphatase by New York surgeons, BENJAMIN S BARRINGER and H O WOODWARD.

1938 The protein nature of renin was suggested by SIR GEORGE W PICKERING, an English professor of medicine, and MYRON PRINZMETAL, an American cardiologist.

1938   The first monograph in pediatric urology was written by MEREDITH CAMPBELL of America.

1938   SANDERS T FRANK born.
An American physician who described oblique fissure of the ear lobe associated with coronary disease, hypertension and diabetes (Frank sign).

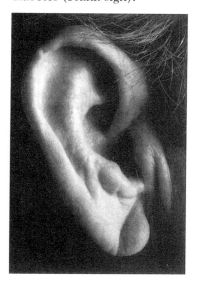

Sanders T Frank described the oblique fissure of the ear

1938   WILLEM JOHAN KOLFF, a Dutch-born American physician and pioneer of the artificial kidney, constructed the first rotating drum artificial kidney, and later developed the artificial kidney (1943) and a heart–lung machine.

1939   The enzymatic nature of renin and its action on angiotonin was demonstrated by EDUARDO BRAUN-MENENDEZ from Buenos Aires and Argentinian Nobel Prize winner, LUIS FREDERICO LELOIR and colleagues.

1939 CHARLES BRENTON HUGGINS, a Canadian-born American surgeon found that cancer cells, as well as the prostate gland, were stimulated by male hormones (androgens). In 1941 he successfully treated bladder cancer with hormones, and developed their use in treating breast cancer. In 1966 he shared the Nobel Prize for his work in cancer research.

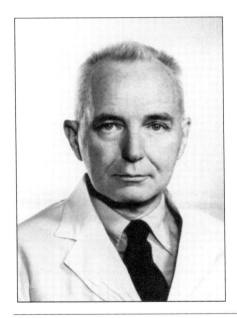

Charles Brenton Huggins
(1901–1997)

1940 Brachial neuritis due to lateral herniation of the cervical intervertebral disc was first described by B STOOKY.

1940 The causative bacteria of rheumatic fever, previously named, *Diplococcus rheumaticus* by FREDERICK JOHN POYNTON and ALEXANDER PAINE, was identified as Streptococcus group A by New York bacteriologist, REBECCA CRAIGHILL LANCEfiELD.

1941 The measurement of 17-ketosteroid levels in urine was introduced as a diagnostic test for hypopituitarism by R FRASER and HOMER SMITH. Smith discovered and used inulin to obtain a precise measure of glomerular filtration rate as inulin is excreted unchanged. He published *Physiology of the Kidney* and *The Kidney: Structure and Function in Health and Disease*.

1941 The Ham test, hemolysis of red cells after incubation with acidified serum, for diagnosis of paroxysmal nocturnal hemoglobinuria, was devised by American physicians, G C HAM and H M HORACK.

1941 J BORNSTEIN and P TREWHELLA demonstrated the phenomenon of insulin resistance.

1943 The first rotating-drum artificial kidney was used to treat a patient by Dutch-born American physician, WILLEM JOHAN KOLFF.

1943 HERBERT FREDERICK TRAUT and American anatomist, GEORGE NICOLAS PAPANICOLAOU, published *The Diagnosis of Uterine Cancer by Vaginal Smear.*

1943 Penicillin was first used in the treatment of syphilis by JOHN FRIEND MAHONEY and colleagues, of the US Public Health Service.

1944 H T J BERK designed the first artificial kidney of therapeutic significance.

1945 The first clear evidence of the causal relationship between renal disease and erythrocytosis was provided by Australian physician, KENNETH FAIRLEY, who described cases caused by renal carcinoma and demonstrated its remission by removing the tumors.

1945 OWEN, an American surgeon, found that non-identical twin calves could tolerate each others' transplanted cells and surmised that sharing the same circulation in the womb had somehow desensitized them to each other.

1946 Norepinephrine was shown to be the main transmitter of sympathetic nerve impulses by Swedish pharmacologist, ULF SVANTE VON EULER, who won the Nobel Prize 24 years later.

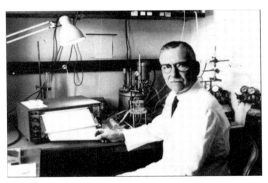

Ulf Svante von Euler (1905–1983)

1946 Nitrofuranotoin, an oral urinary antibacterial compound, was developed from nitrofuran drugs, and introduced by M DODD.

1946 GUIDO FANCONI, a Swiss professor of pediatrics at Zurich, described renal tubular dysfunction (Fanconi syndrome) leading to aminoaciduria and cystic fibrosis of the pancreas.

1946 JACOB FINE used peritoneal irrigation as treatment of acute renal failure.

1948 Nobel laureates, FULLER ALBRIGHT and F C REIFENSTEIN, described renal tubular acidosis causing chronic hyperchloremic acidosis, nephrolithiasis, and recurrent urinary tract infection.

1948 The routine use of rectal biopsy in proctology was established by the English surgeon, WILLIAM BAHALL GABRIEL.

1950 The first suggestion of cardiac output as the primary regulator of renal sodium and water excretion was made by J G BORST and L A deVRIES.

1951 J BORNSTEIN and P TREWHELLA demonstrated the phenomenon of insulin resistance.

1951 An adrenalectomy was successfully performed for breast cancer by American surgeons, CHARLES BRENTON HUGGINS and DAO. HUGGINS pioneered hormonal treatment of cancer, and investigated the physiology of the male urinogenital tract.

1951 Cortisone, the first immunosuppressant, was developed. Eight years later, mercaptopurine and irradiation were used to successfully induce immunological tolerance.

1952 The water excretion test for adrenal function was devised by L J SOFFER and J L GABRILOV.

1952 The sodium-retaining factor in venous blood from the adrenal glands, aldosterone, was identified through chromatography by S A SIMPSON, J F TWIT and P G G BUSH.

1953 The concept of graft versus host reaction in transplantation medicine was put forward by M SIMONSEN.

1953 British biochemist, SIR HANS ADOLF KREBS, and German-born American biochemist, FRITZ ALBERT LIPMANN, shared the Nobel Prize for Physiology or Medicine for their work on the citric acid cycle.

1953 A modification of the percutaneous technique for catheterization of the kidney, allowing the introduction of a catheter of a diameter larger than that of the needle used for initial puncture, was devised by Swedish radiologist, SVEN SELDINGER.

1953 O SPUHLER and H U ZOLLINGER noted the association between prolonged analgesic use and chronic renal failure, analgesic nephropathy.

1953 The Schilling test for vitamin B_{12} absorption by oral administration of radioactive vitamin B_{12} and urinary excretion of radioactivity was studied by American hematologist, ROBERT FREDERICK SCHILLING.

1954 Idiopathic hypercalcemia of childhood was described by I MCQUARRIE.

1954 HAROLD HOPKINS, a British optical physicist, published details of the fiberoptic endoscope in *Nature*.

1954 A successful renal transplant between identical twins was made by American surgeon and pioneer in this field, JOSEPH EDWARD MURRAY and coworkers, at the Peter Bent Brigham Hospital.

1954 Disturbances of pyridoxine metabolism due to isoniazid or isonicotinic acid hydrazide therapy was first demonstrated by J P Biehl and R W Vilter.

1955 Hemolytic uremic syndrome, associated with renal failure, hemolysis and thrombocytopenia, was first described by Swiss pediatrician, C Gasser and coworkers at the University of Zurich.

1955 E H Kass demonstrated the value of 'clean-catch' mid-stream urine for detecting urinary tract infection.

1955 Excessive secretion of aldosterone leading to hypernatremia, hypertension and hypokalemic alkalosis (Conn syndrome) was described by American physician, Jerome William Conn.

1955 J W Cromwell and W L Read were the first to demonstrate that heparization could prevent the formation of minute blood clots; and low-dose heparin treatment for patients at high risk of embolism was introduced in the early 1970s.

1955 Zollinger–Ellison syndrome of recurrent peptic ulceration associated with non-insulin secreting islet cell tumors of the pancreas was described by two American surgeons at Ohio State University, Robert Zollinger and Edwin Ellison.

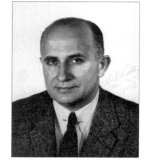

Robert Milton Zollinger
(1903–1992)

1956   With their twin-coiled artificial kidney,
        B WATSCHINGER and WILLEM KOLFF reported two cases of
        uremia treated by hemodialysis and ultrafiltration.

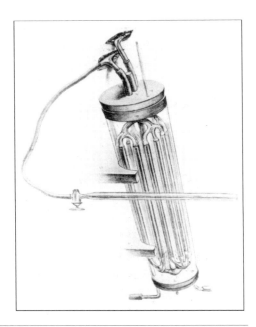

Kolff's first rotating
drum artificial kidney

1956   A sulfonylurea compound (tolbutamide) was introduced as
        treatment in diabetes by HELMUT MASKE of Germany.

1957   The role of the kidney in erythropoiesis was demonstrated by
        L O JACOBSON and coworkers.

1957   A syndrome of inappropriate anti-diuretic hormone
        (ADH) secretion in two patients with bronchogenic
        carcinoma with hyponatremia, inappropriate sodium
        loss and water retention due to ADH, was described by
        American physician, FREDERICK C BARTTER.

1958   Pleural dialysis as a treatment for uremia was introduced by V GORLITZER, B DeMORAIS and J HAMBURGER.

1958   American biochemists and geneticists, GEORGE WELLS BEADLE, JOSHUA LEDERBERG and EDWARD LAURIE TATUM, were awarded the Nobel Prize for Physiology or Medicine for their work on the role of genes in biochemical processes.

1958   Zieve syndrome, jaundice, hyerlipidemia, fatty liver and hemolytic anemia related to alcohol intake, was described by American physician, LESLIE ZIEVE.

1959   Cardiac and renal involvement with pneumonia due to a virus (Lassa fever) was named after Lassa in Nigeria, where the disease was first described.

1959   The first kidney transplant between non-identical twins was successfully carried out at Boston, and for the first time, tissue rejection was successfully treated with drugs.

1959   The first subtotal parathyroidectomy for hyperparathyroidism secondary to uremia and renal failure was performed by S W STANBURY.

1960   Erythrocytosis in polycystic kidneys was first described by C W GURNEY.

1960   The selective uptake of norepinephrine by sympathetic nerves was demonstrated, with the use of radioactive tracers, by JULIUS AXELROD of the American National Institute of Health.

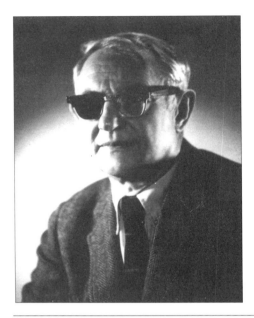

Julius Axelrod
(born 1912)

1960 FULLER ALBRIGHT noted the association between renal calculi and hyperparathyroidism. He is considered the father of endocrinology in America, and described bone change in kidney diseases, osteomalacia of steatorrhea, vitamin D-resistant rickets and the symptomology of Parkinson disease.

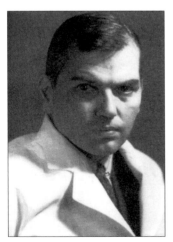

Fuller Albright
(1900–1969)

1961   The first attempt to prepare erythropoietin from renal tissue in vitro was made by Englishman, D G Pennington, who explained its role in the pathogenesis of anemia due to chronic renal failure.

1963   Antilymphocytic serum (ALS), made from animal blood that had been injected previously with human lymphocytes, was shown to prolong survival rates of organ transplants.

1963   Joseph Murray and colleagues at the Brigham Hospital reported on the success of kidney transplants using the immunosuppressive drug, azathioprine.

1963   Hepatitis, encephalopathy and multi-organ failure in children following an acute mild illness (Reye syndrome) was described by an Australian physician of German origin, Ralph Douglas Reye.

1963   Hypoparathyroidism, a condition of hypocalcemia, hyperphosphatemia and radiological bone changes in a girl patient, was described by J M Costello and C E Dent.

1963   Allan Macleod Cormack, a South African-born physicist, developed mathematical principles for the X-ray imaging of 'soft' biological tissue and confirmed its viability experimentally. He showed that by combining X-ray images, it was possible to build up a picture of a slice through soft tissue.

1964   A flexible fiberoptic esophagoscope was described by P A LoPresti and A M Hilmi.

1964   JOHN HOPEWELL and colleagues at the Royal Free Hospital published their results of kidney transplantations using the immunosuppressive drug, 6-mercaptopurine.

1965   S O FREEDMAN and P GOLD demonstrated the presence of tumor-specific antigens in human colonic cancer, through immunological and absorption techniques.

1965   Lupoid hepatitis, active chronic hepatitis accompanied by markers of autoimmune disease, was described by I R MACKAY, S WEIDEN and J HASKER.

1968   American biochemists, ROBERT WILLIAM HOLLEY and MARSHALL WARREN NIRENBERG, and Indian-born American molecular chemist, HAR GOBIND KHORANA, were awarded the Nobel Prize for Physiology or Medicine for their work on the genetic code and amino acid synthesis.

1972   An ultrasonic device to fragment kidney stones without causing bleeding (lithotripter) was invented by two Germans, EISENBERGER and CHAUSSEY in Munich.

1974   Azothioprine, which interferes with cell metabolism, was developed and an antibiotic, cyclosporin, was discovered.

1974   Belgian-born American biologist, ALBERT CLAUDE, English-born Belgian biochemist, CHRISTIAN RENÉ DU DUVE, and Romanian cell biologist, GEORGE EMIL PALADE, were awarded the Nobel Prize for Physiology or Medicine for their work on the substructure and biochemistry of cells.

1977   J F BOREL published his results on organ transplantation using the new immunosuppressant drug, cyclosporin, which markedly increased survival rates.

1977   AXEL ULLRICH published a paper on rat insulin genes and construction of plasmids containing the coding sequences.

1978   HAROLD HOPKINS, an optical physicist, published a chapter on his invention of the modern urological endoscope, a modification of the Leitz cystoscope.

1979   BASIL HIRSCHOWITZ published *A Personal History of the Fiberscope*, and a monograph on its use since his early development of the instrument.

1979   Percutaneous transluminal dilatation of stenozed renal arteries was performed as treatment for renal hypertension by ANDREAS R GRUENTZIG and coworkers.

1980   DAVID A ROBINSON of Manchester identified *Campylobacter jejuni* as a cause of intestinal illness.

1982   JOHN BENJAMIN MURPHY published *Cholecysto-Intestinal , Gastro-Intestinal, Entero-Intestinal Anastomosis, and Approximation without Sutures*. He developed the Murphy kidney punch and Murphy button, a two piece device to make an artificial anastomosis between two hollow abdominal viscera.

1982   Insulin was the first genetically engineered hormone to be approved by the FDA, and marketed by Eli Lilly.

1983 The WHO published results from the Multiple Risk Factor Intervention Trial in which over 50,000 men had been selected and allocated to either intervention or control groups in relation to diet, lifestyle and heart disease in the 1970s. The results showed that death rates from heart disease did not differ between control and intervention groups.

1983 Familial hypertriglyceridemia of autosomal dominant origin was described by H N NEUFIELD and U GOLDBOURT.

1984 The association between hepatitis B surface antigen and hepatocellular carcinoma was observed by ALFRED M PRINCE of the New York Blood Center.

1984 Australian physician, BARRY J MARSHALL, discovered, through self-experimentation, and identified *Helicobacter pylori* as the cause of gastritis and the probable cause of duodenal ulcers. He also noted remission in patients treated with antibiotics.

1986 A tiny television camera was added to the modern laparoscope, making a major advance in keyhole surgery.

1988 Scottish pharmacologist, SIR JAMES WHYTE BLACK, American biochemists, GERTRUDE BELLE ELION and GEORGE HERBERT HITCHINGS were awarded the Nobel Prize for Physiology or Medicine for their work on drugs for heart disease, leukemia, the anti-viral drug, acyclovir, and the anti-AIDS drug, zidovudine.

1990 THOMAS STARZL of the Veterans' Administration Hospital in Colorado published a survey of long-term survival of renal homograft patients, half of whom had survived with immunosuppressive and steroid anti-rejection drugs.

1992 American biochemists, EDMOND HENRI FISCHER and EDWIN GERHARD KREBS were awarded the Nobel Prize for Physiology or Medicine for their work on the role of phosphorylation–dephosphorylation in activation of glycogen phosphorylase by adenylic acid.

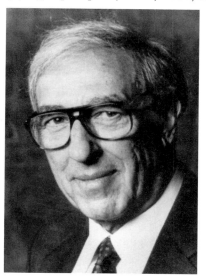

Edmond Henri Fischer
(born 1920)

1995 G B CLEMENTS and colleagues showed that the coxsackie virus attacks insulin-producing cells in the pancreas and can lead to childhood diabetes.

1997 A virus was proposed as a cause of insulin-dependent type-1 diabetes by BERNARD CONRAD and colleagues at the University of Geneva.

1999 Trials begin of the first drug, developed in Canada, against the killer bacterium, *E. coli* 0157, that causes hemolytic uremic syndrome and kidney damage.

1999 DAVID HUMES and colleagues at the University of Michigan develop an artificial kidney lined with living kidney cells which puts back essential molecules from the urine.

1999 A vaccine trial against persistent bladder and urinary tract infections, caused by *Escherichia coli*, begins.

1999 Cyclosporin is linked to the spread of cancers by MINORU HOJO of Cornell University.

1999 GÜNTER BLOBEL of the Rockefeller University in New York was awarded the Nobel Prize for Physiology or Medicine for his discovery that proteins have intrinsic signals that govern their transport and localization in the cell. This research aids our understanding of the molecular mechanisms involved in many genetic diseases, such as cystic fibrosis or hyperoxaluria, and of the functioning of the immune system.